NEW PERSPECTIVES ON MUTUAL DEPENDENCY IN CARE-GIVING

The book was published thanks to the institutional support for the development of the Office for Population Studies, Faculty of Social Studies, Masaryk University.

New Perspectives on Mutual Dependency in Care-Giving

ADÉLA SOURALOVÁ
Masaryk University, Czech Republic

Routledge
Taylor & Francis Group
LONDON AND NEW YORK

First published 2015 by Ashgate Publishing

Published 2016 by Routledge
2 Park Square, Milton Park, Abingdon, Oxon OX14 4RN
711 Third Avenue, New York, NY 10017, USA

Routledge is an imprint of the Taylor & Francis Group, an informa business

British Library Cataloguing in Publication Data
A catalogue record for this book is available from the British Library

The Library of Congress has cataloged the printed edition as follows:
Souralová, Adéla.
New perspectives on mutual dependency in care-giving / by Adéla Souralová.
pages cm
Includes bibliographical references and index.
ISBN 978-1-4724-5666-3 (hardback)
1. Caregivers. 2. Helping behavior. I. Title.
HM1146.S68 2015
362'.0425--dc23

2015008100

ISBN: 9781472456663 (hbk)

Contents

List of Figures and Tables

Figures

Tables

Appendices

Acknowledgements

This book has been conceived and developed over a long period of time, and could never been completed without the help and support of number of people. Most obviously, I would like to thank everyone who gave their time to talk to me: the second generation Vietnamese children who took me to their childhood; their mothers who—despite their time-consuming jobs—found the opportunity to talk about their post-migratory lives; and the Czech nannies who quite openly spoke about the role of care-giving in their lives. Their willingness to speak about very private topics was invaluable.

A number of academic colleagues have helped and encouraged me. Professor Steven Saxonberg was my PhD supervisor and source of help and support throughout the writing of my PhD thesis, which forms the basis of this book. Professor Lise Widding Isaksen reviewed the PhD thesis and encouraged me to share my research findings with the international research community. Dr Martin Kreidl suggested publishing my dissertation as a book, and Professor Ladislav Rabušic helped me realize this idea by providing me with a one-year publishing grant at the Office for Population Studies. This book was published thanks to the institutional support for the development of the Office for Population Studies, Faculty of Social Studies, Masaryk University in Brno. I would also like to thank the Jan Hus Educational Foundation for the scholarship it awarded me, and which provided appreciable financial aid for undertaking my research. I am also deeply grateful to Judy Mayers, who did the English language editing of this book.

This book would also never have been completed without the warm support of my friends who were willing to listen to my "stories from the field." Notably, I want to thank Denisa Sedláčková for so many hours spent discussing the emerging text. I also want to thank Eva Šlesingerová, my friend and colleague from Social Anthropology at the Faculty of Social Studies, who has been supporting me since the start of my academic career, and who has always believed in what I do and how I do it.

I dedicate this book to two women who shaped my personality, both as a human being and as a researcher and analyst: my mother, Věra Souralová, and my grandmother, Anna Souralová. In the spring of 2012, my grandma's age did not allow her to continue living alone in her house. I started living there with her and caring for her. Our relationship had always been very warm and close. However, the experience of living with my grandmother made our relationship even warmer and closer—we became mutually dependent on each other. It was a time when I was finishing the interviews with the children of Vietnamese immigrants—who often develop deep emotional ties with their Czech grandmothers—and interviews with these Czech grandmothers—who take care of their Vietnamese grandchildren, often with deep affection. When listening to their stories, I felt myself moving back to my own childhood and forward again to the present. Like them, I was the child of a working mother. And like several of them, I had warm relations with my grandma, who had always taken care of me. This close relationship continued, despite the fact our roles had changed over the last few years, as it was I who became her care provider. These two experiences lit my way as a researcher and analyst from the time of the initial definition of research objectives, to the time of the final analysis and writing. Thank you, mum and grandma, for having always supported me, believed in me, and done what was best for me, even though it was not always easy.

Chapter 1
Introduction: "Where do the Children Play?"

Ms. Pham is a 25-year-old Vietnamese immigrant woman who has one 3-year-old daughter named Than. She came to the Czech Republic eight years ago and now works in the immigrant economy as an entrepreneur, the owner of a clothing shop. When her daughter was 8 months old, Ms. Pham started working 10 hours a day. Because of her incorporation into the labour market she had to look for another woman to care for little Than. Ms. Brhlíková is a 55-year-old Czech woman. She has three adult children of her own with whom she spent 12 years on parental leave. Now she is a pensioner informally working for Ms. Pham. She does care-giving work for little Than with whom she spends five days per week, from morning to evening. Than calls her "grandma" and Ms. Brhlíková feels happy, because she does not have grandchildren yet. These women of three generations are part of the global division of reproductive labour, but their situation differs from that of Filipina domestic workers in the USA, Polish domestic workers in Germany, or Czech au pairs in the UK.

This book focuses on the experiences of Vietnamese immigrant women who hire Czech nannies (such as Ms. Pham), the experiences of Czech women who work as nannies for Vietnamese immigrant families (as Ms. Brhlíková) and finally the experiences of second generation immigrant children who are brought up by Czech nannies. It looks into the issue of care work, migration and family relations. During the last two decades, an increasing number of households employed a care/domestic worker. Over decade ago, the *National Survey of America's Families* showed that 4 percent of the children of immigrants under the age of three were cared for by nannies/babysitters (compared to 6 percent for children of US-born citizens; Matthews and Ewen, 2006). The increasing number of households that employ care workers has led to a boom in the research on this topic (Sarti, 2014). However, these studies focused on the 6 percent of households, comprised of non-migrant (and usually well-off, middle-class) families that hire migrant care/domestic workers (Parreñas, 2001; Anderson, 2000; Momsen, 1999; Lutz, 2008; 2011; Hondagneu-Sotelo, 2001; Macdonald, 2010; Chang, 2000; Lan, 2006; Isaksen, 2010, and so on). Thus, they have neglected the 4 percent of immigrant households which hire care workers. This is especially strange given the growing literature on second generation immigrant children. Hardly any studies have explored the care strategies of working immigrant parents and the consequences for the lives of their children. Thus, in recent decades, two parallel scholarly trends have developed in the international scientific discourse: scholarship on care work and scholarship on second generation immigrant children.

This book contributes to these two scholarly traditions by being the first academic study on children of immigrants who are raised by native nannies. Not only does this study make an important empirical contribution to the scientific discourse, it also contributes methodological and conceptual innovations. The book develops further the discussion on care work and brings new perspectives to the research agenda. It follows three steps:

1. Making visible the experience of immigrant families hiring the nannies (empirical innovation);
2. Adding a new perspective—the perspective of the children (methodological innovation); and
3. Taking as its starting point the concept and phenomenon of 'mutual dependency' (theoretical innovation).

By making immigrant care work demanders visible, bringing children into the care work research, and proposing the notion of mutual dependency as a useful tool in analyzing care work relationships, this book offers a new perspective on general care work theory and research. It encourages scholars to re-think the current conceptual frameworks built upon the experiences of immigrant domestic workers and middle-class families.

With its empirical innovation and *focus on immigrant families*, this book draws upon Asian immigrants' experience with care-giving and the delegation of care work. Asian migrants are expanding their participation in the global economy in many parts of the world. The second generation of Asian immigrants are usually taken as an example of successful assimilation (especially in terms of their educational achievements). Meanwhile their parents are portrayed as hard workers in businesses, who make sacrifices in their private lives to succeed in a new country in order to provide their children with sufficient economic capital (Song, 1999). It is, therefore, quite logical to ask "where do the children play?" and who cares for them while their parents care about breadwinning. Asking this question enables us to reveal a side of the lives of Asian immigrants that has so far been hidden. Making visible the immigrant families that recruit nannies for their children means making visible the links between care-giving and integration, between migration and welfare regimes, as well as tensions between care ideologies and mothering strategies in post-migratory context.

The second step brings the methodological innovation—*the shift toward the children's perspective*. The book is the first sociological study on care work that includes the perspective of children that have (had) nannies taking care of them. When asking "where do the children play?" while their parents work, it pays particular attention to the incorporation of such children into research on care work. In doing so, it synthesizes three perspectives: care workers, care demanders, and care receivers. In her analysis of the "nanny" question in feminism, Joan C. Tronto (2002) distinguishes three perspectives for understanding paid childcare: the perspective of the nanny, of the parents, and of the child. However, the general scholarship on domestic work provides no clue as to how children see this constellation of relationships. Most research on the child's perspective focuses on children left behind in their home countries, while their mothers come to Western countries to take care of children there, who enjoy an emotional surplus (Romero, 1997; Parreñas, 2005). The research on delegated care work has not paid much attention to the perspective of children who are *currently* being looked after by nannies, or adults who previously had been looked after by nannies. The reason for this neglect may be concern for ethical issues related to doing research on children. It may also be due to the assumption that children are passive objects in the social structure, and that their perspective can only be mediated by adults (Prout and James, 1997). However, during the last three decades—a period coincidentally marked by a boom in literature on domestic/care work—a new approach to children in social science research has been developing. Children are starting to be taken seriously as social actors with their own viewpoint and agency. The change of paradigm, it seems anyway, has had no impact on care work research.

And last but not least, this book aims to contribute to our understanding of care work by *further developing a concept of mutual dependency*. Many scholars have seen care-giving relationships as being based on mutual dependency or interdependency (Glenn, 1992; Lutz, 2008; 2011; Andall, 2003). The extensively cited notions of the "global care chain" (Hochschild, 2000) or "international division of reproductive labor" (Parreñas, 2001) prepared the ground for the analysis of global interdependencies in several domains. My approach takes a further step by taking mutual dependency as a starting point for the analysis of all relationships. I argue that beyond the emergence of these new relationships lies the need of each participant for all the other participants—the need of families for nannies, and the need of nannies for families (children and parents). These needs are met in the daily practice of care-giving, and lead to the emergence of interdependencies between mothers and nannies and nannies and children. Hence, I start with the main question "What is the character of the relationships among parents, nannies and children?" Then I focus on what kind of meanings mothers, nannies, and children give to paid care-giving, and what kind of affinities, cooperation, or tensions and contradictions emerge in the paid childcare relationship between nannies, mothers, and their children.

1.1 Seeing Paid Childcare with Children's Eyes

In this book I make an argument for incorporating children into research on delegated childcare. Only when incorporating the perspective of children, can we see the mutuality in care work—mutual reciprocal giving and receiving (not only in economic terms but above all in terms of emotionality, intimacy, or support). So far, the scholars have often asked "Who takes care of the maid's children" (to borrow the title of Romero's article; Romero, 1997, see also Hondagneu-

Sotelo and Avila, 1997) and described how the maid's children learn from early childhood about unequal opportunities and structural hierarchies. Similarly, the children benefiting from these inequalities receive the opposite lesson, as summed up by Tronto (2002, p.40): "Children may well come to expect that other people, regardless of their connection to them, will always be available to meet their needs. They may come to treat people as merely means, and not as ends in themselves." The list of "mays" in children's lives is concluded by Tronto's condemnation of paid childcare, which she believes makes the creation of democratic citizens impossible, as children cared for by servants witness "the arbitrary and capricious interaction of parents and servants, or if they are permitted to treat domestic servants in a similar manner" (*ibid.*).

Surprisingly, the research on delegated care work has not paid much attention to the perspective of cared-for children: either of children *currently* being looked after by nannies, or of adults with the *past* experience of being raised by nannies Addressing the children's perspective on delegated childcare is not just to add and stir in *another* perspective to the already-established framework dealing with the perspectives of employers and employees, but rather to re-think the grounds of research on care work. Within the new sociology of childhood paradigm, children are able to construct their own identities, select the influences of socialization, and create their own perspectives on social phenomena, processes, and institutions (Prout and James, 1997). Using the social construction approach, sociologists attempt to include children's agency to interpret children's lives (Prout and James, 1997; Jenks, 2004; Qvortrup, 1993). As Alan Prout and Allison James (1997, p.8) described one of the features of the paradigm which is important for my analysis: "Children are and must be seen as active in the construction and determination of their own social lives, the lives of those around them and of the societies in which they live. Children are not just the passive subjects of the social structures and processes." Looking at how children of Vietnamese parents brought up by Czech nannies construct their identities, make sense of their lives and intervene in the lives of others, this book deals with how children understand their roles *as children* (*vis-à-vis* parents), as *cared-for children* (*vis-à-vis* nannies), and as Czech or Vietnamese (perception of *ethnic identities*). There are at least three reasons why it is important to look into the children's perspective on delegated care-giving: First, it sheds new light on how care-giving establishes ties of intimacy and emotionality. Second, it provides a reconsideration of what motherhood means and how it should be performed. And third, it reveals how care-giving is fundamentally a bonding activity which leads to the creation of kinship ties.

Focusing on children's perspectives illuminates the character of *intimacy and emotionality* in delegated childcare. Research that includes the perspective of cared-for children can move beyond the basic assumption that paid care work is by nature an exploitative relationship between two women. It is an *employment* relationship between employer and employee in which the content is carried out between nanny and child. The dynamic of the latter relationship (nanny-child) can differ to a great extent from that of the former relationship (employer-employee), which makes childcare work both ambiguous and paradoxical. As Uttal and Tuominen (1999, p.776, italics added) argue: "the paradoxical character of paid childcare work combines the structural inequality of employer-employee relations with the potential for the work to be emotionally significant to the *workers* and to *those who hire the workers*."

On the one hand—between employers and employees—care work relationships are filled with asymmetries and hierarchies, domination and subordination. There are many studies that capture the intimate negotiations of power relations and asymmetries in daily activities such as serving food, accommodation, and particular childcare tasks (from feeding and changing diapers to bed time rituals), or communication between employer, employee and child (Anderson, 2000; Rollins, 1985; Hondagneu-Sotelo, 2001; Constable, 1997; Búriková and Miller, 2010). Social, ethnic, and class inequalities are omnipresent in many domains of both private and public life, and crystallize in the mother-nanny relationship (Macdonald, 2010). That is why one of the critical issues that has been extensively discussed is that of exploitation. Some scholars have used the framework of slavery to describe new forms of inequalities in domestic work that arise when one person pays while another is paid (Anderson, 2000; Apitzsch, 2007). A domestic worker becomes a commodity (for commodification see Anderson, 2000; 2003) that can be bought, similar to the process of First World exploitation of Third World resources. In this respect, as Bridget Anderson in her influential book argues, "the employer is buying the power to command, not the property in the person, but the whole person" (Anderson, 2000, p.113). However, as the empirical data on domestic work has demonstrated, relations between employers and employees are far more complex (Lutz, 2011), and the inequalities and asymmetries show their contradictory nature when focusing on the micropolitics of care work.

On the other hand, between nannies and children, care work establishes radically different set of ties—those based on emotional exchange and sharing intimacy. Since care and emotions are inseparably linked, care work is without any doubt an example of what Hochschild (1983) calls "emotional labor." Developing the concept of "feeling rules," she sets the conceptual framework for understanding the nature of the commercialization of feelings. Her contribution was further elaborated by Margaret K. Nelson (1990), who discusses the character of "feeling rules" within childcare. Day care providers, according to Nelson, have to deal with the discrepancy between "being like mother" and "being mother." Both mothers and care workers thus have to negotiate the emotional dilemma inherent in delegated childcare. Mothers want nannies to love their children so that they (the mothers) can work tranquilly outside the home, but at the same time they feel uncomfortable if the children develop strong attachments to nannies or even confuse the nannies for their mothers (Lan, 2006). Nannies, at the same time, must manage their own feelings toward the children, and such negotiations create tensions between feeling too much and feeling too little in order to protect themselves from "harm" (typically the sense of loss and pain caused by leaving the family; Nelson, 1990). The central "feeling rule" that Nelson defines is that of "detached attachment," wherein the nannies should like the children they take care of enough, but not too much (similarly, see Macdonald, 1998).

This is what we know about how nannies negotiate their ties to children. However, we do not know much about how children respond to the above-addressed attachments and emotions they receive from nannies. According to Hochschild (2002a), these children are the most privileged in the care chain (contrary to the children of nannies who are left behind), because they enjoy love both from their mothers as well as from other children's mothers—their nannies. While children of nannies are "forced to learn early on that they have to endure the difficulties of life" (Tronto, 2002, p.40; see also Romero, 1992), children cared for by nannies "may come to treat people as merely means, and not as ends in themselves" (*ibid.*). Are the children cared for by nannies the winners in the global emotional battle? What is the nature of their ties with nannies? Children's relationship to nannies should supposedly be less marked by the employment logic than their mothers (mothers buy the childcare service, not the children). The children are *recipients* of care and emotions from nannies, yet they are also active participants in this relationship, and contribute to the emotional exchange with nannies. When we include the perspective of children, childcare work appears to be an emotional activity that requires and generates mutual emotional attachment and investment. Using the concept of "gift" developed by Marcel Mauss (1990 [1922]), we can see that care-giving entails emotions giving, receiving, and reciprocating (Souralová, 2015).

The second reason for incorporating children into research on delegated care-giving is because children actively *make sense of the role of care-giving in defining motherhood.* We know quite a lot about how mothers and nannies negotiate motherhood when childcare is delegated. For example, in her prominent book *Global Cinderellas: Migrant Domestics and Newly Rich Employers in Taiwan*, Pei-Chia Lan (2006) analyses how employers maintain a stratified division of motherhood by marking boundaries between themselves—the biological, permanent mothers—and the nannies who do the substitute mothering. When balancing the emotions of jealousy and deprivation, mothers turn to "mother-only" tasks and strategically "ethnicize" their motherhood. Mothers accentuate some of the components of mothering based on the common language or culture a child shares with the mother and not with a (foreign-born) nanny. One mother interviewed by Lan talked about reading books and telling stories. By making ethnicity part of the bedtime routine, mothers draw boundaries between themselves and their nannies, and highlight the primacy of their relationship with their children, for whom they—the mothers—remain "the rock-steady center" (Macdonald, 2010, p.76). Nannies also distinguish themselves from the mothers—or more precisely, from the way the mothers perform their mothering. Several scholars have demonstrated that mothers participating in the labour market and/or who hire a nanny, have to deal with others' judgments and as well as their own feelings about leaving the child (Arendell, 2000; Walzer, 1997, etc.). Uttal (1993 in Uttal and Tuominen, 1999) found in her research that some care-givers use moral hierarchies—judgments about a mother's mothering—to define themselves as superior to mothers. Simply put, both mothers and nannies draw upon their own subjective definitions of "good motherhood" (Arendell, 2000; Liamputtong, 2006) and apply them in the daily practice of their care-giving and mothering.

How do children subjected to two different forms of care-giving—performed by two women usually from radically different (socio-economic, cultural, or ethnic) backgrounds—perceive care-giving and mothering? Do they judge their mothers as the nannies do? Or do they influence mothers' mothering and make boundaries between motherhood and paid care-giving? What differences do they find between mothers' care-giving and nannies' care-giving? How do they define "good motherhood"? As studies of children left behind by transnational mothers demonstrate, the children perceive changing family relations and make sense of what family and motherhood means (Madianou and Miller, 2012; Parreñas, 2005). It is clear that children are able to distinguish between different strategies of care-giving and upbringing, and to reflect on their positive and negative sides as well as their impact on relationship formation. In addition, answering the above questions may also reveal definitions of childhood—both in the sense of a phase in the life cycle, and in the sense of being a daughter or son.

In the case of immigrant families, the delegation of care-giving impacts post-migratory settlement and intergenerational relations. It has been extensively discussed that the role of mothers in raising second generation immigrant children is crucial. As Umut Erel (2009, p.111) concludes, "in acculturation theories of migration, women, because of their familial role, are considered to be the bearers of 'the more originary type of the culture of origin.'" As the possessors of "traditional Vietnameseness," mothers are seen as passing the culture down to children in the process of care-giving. The question that emerges here is, what happens when the mother does not play her care-giving role in the face-to-face care scenario? Such a model of a parent-child relationship further complicates already-complicated intergenerational ties seen in terms of an "intergenerational gap" (Kibria, 1993; 2002). In her analysis of second-generation Chinese and Korean American identities, Nazli Kibria (2002, p.41) observes that "the theme of culture clashes with parents was quite clearly an important one in the childhood memories of my informants." How are culture clashes with parents contextualized in the delegated childcare relationship? How do children construct their ethnic identities and their Vietnameseness when it is the Czech culture which is passed down to them during care-giving?

And third, children may provide us with insight into how care-giving operates as a *bonding activity*, connecting people (and families) into a kinship network and making them relatives. The emergence of so-called fictive kinship (false kinship or pseudo-family relations, respectively) has been acknowledged in the literature on domestic/care work (Maroufof, 2013; Gregson and Lowe, 1994; Hardin, 2008; Karner, 1998; Búriková and Miller, 2010) as well as in migration research focusing on shifts in family arrangements and ideologies in the post-migratory context (Ebaugh and Curry, 2000; Foner, 1997). For the first research topic the adjective "fictive" is used to demonstrate the falseness of the relationship, which is marked by exploitation. For the second part of the research "fictive" is recalled to describe "a relationship based not on blood or marriage, but either on religious rituals or close friendship ties, that replicates many of the rights and obligations usually associated with family ties" (Ebaugh and Curry, 2000, p.189). Here "fictive" stands in contrast to the "real" and "biological." Put in the post-migratory context, Nancy Foner (1997, p.969) describes how "the absence of immigrants' close kin in the new setting creates the need to improvise new arrangements, a reason why "fictive kin" are common in immigrant communities and why men sometimes find themselves filling in as helpmates to their wives in childcare and other household tasks."

In this book, I do not use the term "fictive kinship," despite the fact that it may fit into the definitions proposed both by Ebaugh and Curry, and by Foner because its employment necessarily poses the question of what real kinship is, and leads us back to the old discussion about the nature of kinship ties—whether the basis for kinship ties are biogenetic or social. In addition, authors such as Janet Carsten (2004, p.146) question the authorship of the term "fictive": "If, in this case, what anthropologists have been used to describing as 'fictive' kinship is asserted to be just as real as 'true' kinship (…) then whose fiction is it?" In this regard, the fiction of fictive kinship is based on an analytic strategy that asserts the primacy of biology (Carsten, 2004; Howell, 2003). For this reason I analyze ties between nannies and children by turning to the modern anthropological theory of kinship that emphasizes the formative role of care in maintaining and reproducing kinship/family ties, and defining what a family is, who is included, and who is not. Ever since the 1970s, when the definition of kinship was unbiologicized (Schneider, 1984), scholarship on the issue has shown that ideas about the family are formed not on the basis of what is given, but on what is done. It was anthropologists of adoption, in particular, who shed light on the process of *becoming* relatives. I am inspired above all by Signe Howell (2003), who has developed the concept of kinning to describe the way an adopted child becomes part of the adopting parents' kin. Based on empirical material obtained from a study of transnational adoption in Norway, Howell defines kinning as "the process by which a foetus or new-born child (or a previously unconnected person) is brought into a significant and permanent relationship with a group of people that is expressed in a kin idiom" (Howell, 2003, p.465). In her view, kinship is "something that is necessarily achieved in and through relationships with others" (*ibid.*, p.468). As with other scholars emphasizing the performative definition of kinship (Sahlins, 2011), the main argument here is that kinship ties do not exist *a priori*, but are negotiated on a daily basis through diverse activities, with care-giving being the most significant of those activities.

Kinship ties usually serve (immigrant) children as a basis for the definition of home (Boehm, 2012). If home is defined through family and kinship ties, and kinship ties are created in the process of caring, how do children of Vietnamese parents cared for by Czech nannies comprehend what is family, kinship, and home(land)? Many scholars have dealt with the question of what second generation immigrants that never or rarely visit their parents' country of origin consider to be their home and homeland (Espiritu, 2003; collection edited by Levitt and Walters, 2002; and so on). In this context, Diane Wolf (2002) develops the concept of "emotional transnationalism," while Yen Le Espiritu (2003) offers the notion of "symbolic transnationalism." Both authors refer to the imaginaries of homeland which are shaped, inter alia, by the person's position in family/kinship network. As Wolf (2002, p.258) argues, emotional transnationalism "situates them between different generational and locational points of reference, both real and the imagined—their parents,' sometimes also their grandparents' and other relatives,' and their own." The author uses this terminology to illustrate the "fluid movement back and forth" and the process of establishing identities deeply connected to the ancestors' homeland (in this case the Philippines). Her contribution makes evident that ethnic identities are formed "not simply on one place," but that this process includes interactions with the Philippines (*ibid.*). The character of these interactions is already apparent in the adjective "emotional," or "symbolic"; and as Tran and Espiritu (2002, p.369) emphasizes, these adjectives do not mean that the interactions take place at the literal level. Rather they operate on the level of imagination, shared memory, and "inventions of traditions"; hence they conceive of their homeland "not only as a physical place that immigrants and their children return to for visits but also as a concept and a desire—a place to return to through the imagination."

When considering children's perceptions and thoughts about their homeland, the book takes the analytical approach that the homeland is something shaped in the process of imagination (Rushdie, 1992; Said, 1984). The homeland can be returned to through imagination and memories, not only by physical return visits. Ketu Katrak (1996, p.201 in Tran and Espiritu, 2002, p.369) speaks of the "simultaneity of geography (…) the possibility of living here in body and elsewhere in mind and imagination." In Chapter 6 of this book I look into how second generation Vietnamese children imagine their homeland and how these imaginations are closely connected to their understanding of kinship ties.

1.2 Study Design: Researching Mother-Nanny-Child Triangle

The purpose of this research project was to analyze three differing but essentially connected perspectives and experiences within delegated childcare—those of mothers, nannies and children. The formulation of my research objectives began with my interest in Vietnamese children that have had the experience of being cared for by Czech nannies. From this initial starting point it became apparent that I would be interested not only in current paid care-giving, but above all in the consequences and outcomes of former paid care-giving. I aimed at examining the *dynamics* of these relationships, and their *continuity* and changeability over the life course of the people in the sample. Paid care-giving is inevitably a time-bounded activity, meaning that it establishes a set of responsibilities and relationships that change over the years the children are growing up, and end once children achieve self-sufficiency and no longer depend on nannies and mothers. I therefore I directed my research towards the examination of two forms of relationships: (1) relationships that are created during the current paid care-giving, and (2) relationships that are maintained and reproduced when the paid care-giving terminates.

In order to trace these two forms of relationships, I had to precisely define my sampling design. All sampling in qualitative research may be encompassed under the broad umbrella term of *purposeful sampling* (Patton, 1990). Purposeful sample provides "a clear criterion and rationale for the selection of participants," as Ezzy (2002, p.74) writes, accentuating that "the reasons for the sample are clearly related to the research question" (*ibid.*). With regard to this, I created a list of criteria for my sample in pursuit of my main objectives. These criteria were specific for each of the target groups; however, the essential condition was that all of my interviewees must have been "in contact" with a care-giver (in the case of mothers and children) or cared-for child (in the case of nannies).

Data collection took place between April 2010 and November 2012, when I conducted interviews with 57 interviewees: nannies (15), children (20) and mothers (15), and gatekeepers (7). Below I submit a basic description of my interviewees, as well as a description of the actors included in the triangle of relationships between mothers, children, and nannies.

The interviews with *children* focused on recollections of childhood and a description of their current relationship to the nanny. Therefore, in the selection of child interviewees I took into account three criteria. The first criterion, was that the children are still in touch with their nannies. I did not specify in detail what level of intensity "being in contact" meant, because I expected that the intensity of contact would change over the course of the children's and nannies' lives. However, I excluded potential interviewees that reported having had a nanny but did not remember anything about her, and those that had not had further relations with the nanny once paid care-giving terminated. In my sample, I had children whose ties to their nannies varied from almost daily contact, to occasional visits.

The second criterion was the child interviewees' age, which I limited to 16–25 years. I did this in view of the data collection method—in-depth interviews—and my interest in capturing the *long-term* aspect of the children-nanny relationship. I also decided on these age limits because I assumed that young people at this age think a great deal about their ties with parents, their ethnic identities, and about their sense of belonging—both in relation to their past and to their future—such as when dealing with their partner's lives and anticipating their own family trajectories.

The third criterion was place of birth. My goal was to carry out interviews with children who were born in the Czech Republic (10 of my interviewees), as well as with children who came with or later joined their parents in the Czech Republic at the age of 7 or younger (10 of my interviewees). According to the standard classification of immigrant children (Levitt, 2002; Oropesa and Landale, 1997), my informants would be called "second generation" (born in the Czech

Republic), 1.75 generation (born in Vietnam and coming to the Czech Republic at the age of five or younger), and 1.5 generation (born in Vietnam and coming to the Czech Republic at ages six to twelve). In this book, I call all of my child interviewees "second generation," and do not distinguish among them, unless it is relevant for the analysis. I assumed the criterion of place of birth would be important (and it proved itself to be) when considering the character of the nanny-child relationship, its framing in the kinship idiom, and its role in the conception of belonging (Chapter 6).

In my sample of *mother-interviewees*, there were mothers currently employing nannies, as well as mothers who had employed nannies in the past. In addition to the second model, the mothers or their children must have been in touch at least with one of the nannies (if they had more than one nanny).

The mothers I met during the research varied widely, both in their experience of immigration, as well as (to a lesser extent) their current situation (employment and type of residence). The parents arrived to the country between the 1980s (the era of socialist cooperation between Czechoslovakia and Vietnam; see below) and 2005. A large proportion of my interviewees came to the Czech Republic because they already had some relatives here. A frequent pattern was that the man came in the 1980s to study, returned to Vietnam where he married, and then came back to the Czech Republic with his wife (and children). The status of the parents depends on when they arrived: most of them have permanent residence; temporary residence is an exception. None of my mother-interviewees had Czech citizenship. They did not want it, and they assumed they would be returning to Vietnam once their children were grown and financially secure.

I intentionally did not carry out any interviews with fathers as my analytical strategy was to trace the relationships among women. To understand the two levels of the mother-nanny relationship—one based on the ethnic logic of the relationship between *Vietnamese* employer and *Czech* employee, the second based on the employment logic of the relationship between Vietnamese *employer* and Czech *employee*. At the same time, as became obvious during the collection of data, it was usually women who were responsible for the delegation of childcare: it was the woman's decision to return to work which led to the decision to hire a nanny, and it was the mothers (not the fathers) who were stigmatized by others.

I carried out 17 interviews with a total of 15 *nannies* (Ms. Brhlíková and Ms. Křepelková were interviewed twice, first in 2010, and again in 2011). Following the logic outlined above, the interviewees were either currently employed as nannies, or had been employed as nannies in the past, and were still in touch with the families (usually the children) they had looked after.

All of the nannies with one exception shared a basic characteristic: they all were dependent on the state social welfare system. This fact is key to understanding the entire relationship between the Vietnamese families and the Czech nannies. As to family status, four of the women lived by themselves (either divorced or widowed), and were thus the sole breadwinners in their household. Most of my nanny-interviewees worked in one family. If they worked in more than one family, the nanny was employed *subsequently* in these families, not simultaneously. When I was finishing my research, I learned that a new model of delegated childcare had arrived in the Vietnamese "community": one Czech woman taking care of more than one child from more than one family. This model was not included in my sample, and therefore the nannies whom I interviewed always worked as one nanny for one family/child.

My initial thought was to elaborate on the particular case studies of mother-child-nanny and mother-nanny relationships. This meant interviewing all two/three actors of one dyad/triad, and analyzing it as a unit of relations, practices and meanings. However, this aim was hard to accomplish due to my often limited access to potential interviewees. During my research I never had problems contacting child interviewees. However I had much greater difficulty contacting nannies, and found it nearly impossible to get in touch with mothers. If I had relied exclusively on the above dyads/triads, my research would have taken longer, and would have been deprived of interviews with children who provided me with rich data and colourful stories, but whose mothers or nannies did not agree to be interviewed. Still, during the interviews I had the chance to interview two dyads: Ms. Pham—Ms. Brhlíková, and Ms. Ho—Ms. Dudková, and two triads: Ms. Truong—Mihn—Ms. Kosová, Ms. Ngo—Anh—Ms. Andulková.

Summarizing the characteristics of the sample with regard to my research objectives, the interviewees selected by the above-specified criteria provided me with the following kinds of interpretations in the interviews:

1. relationships that are created during the current paid care-giving: *recollections* of former care-giving given by 20 child interviewees, seven mother-interviewees, eight nanny-interviewees, and *delineations* of current care-giving given by eight mother-interviewees, seven nanny-interviewees; and
2. relationships that are maintained and reproduced when the paid care-giving terminates: *delineations* of current relationships given by 20 child interviewees, seven mother-interviewees, eight nanny-interviewees.

I recruited my informants using the *snowball sampling method.* Most of the first contacts took place through the second generation: I addressed university students with the question of whether they had had a Czech nanny or knew someone that had. To avoid having all my informants belong to the same network, I did not rely on a single entrance to the community of my informants, but on several of them. Relying on only one gatekeeper would have been impossible, as the chain established by one interviewee-gatekeeper was soon broken, and hence did not provide me with a rich source of data.

It was usually through the child interviewees that I established contact with the nannies and parents. In light of the intimate character of the entire study, I was forced to rely on recommendations to find people suitable for the research, and to rely even more on *their recommendation of me* as a person that could be trusted. This was especially true with the Vietnamese mothers, whom it was not possible to contact ad hoc "through the market" (so to speak), and for whom I was obliged to rely on persons "inside." This recommendation was a very helpful way of overcoming the a priori mistrust on the part of my informants. This mistrust originates from the fact that care is considered a private matter—hidden from the eyes of public (and also from the researcher's)—and from the basic characteristic of the care arrangement—that caring takes place in the irregular labour market. This was the first but not last obstacle that I had to deal with when contacting my informants. Second, when I searched for Vietnamese parents who were paying Czech nannies, I encountered the problem of their intensive labour market participation. Paradoxically I discovered, without doing any interviews, one of the main features of their life and the reason why they hire Czech nannies. The third obstacle I encountered—and which also tells a lot about Vietnamese immigrant life—was the language barrier. Since I do not speak Vietnamese, I had to conduct all the interviews in Czech. However, even though some parents were willing to talk with me, their poor knowledge of Czech (and my total ignorance of Vietnamese) made the interviews impossible without the help of interpreters.

Conducting interviews with the help of an *interpreter* was the greatest challenge to my research. For a long time interpreters have been invisible figures in the social science research process. This invisibility was considered necessary for maintaining "objectivity" and eliminating "bias" in qualitative research. The role of the interpreter had to be minimized, reduced to a neutral mouthpiece, as Temple and Edwards (2002) have shown. The dominant image of the interpreter was "a conduit linking the interviewer with the interviewee, and is ideally a neutral party who should neither add nor subtract from what the primary parties communicate to each other" (Freed, 1988, p.316).

A reflexive turn in the social sciences brought new sensitivity to questions of power in the research process, and the "positionality" of the researcher *vis-à-vis* the researched, as well as new recognition of the role of interpreters in the research process. Now recognized as a key link in research practice, interpreters came to be identified as *active* participants, with their own assumptions about the research being conducted. Several authors have demonstrated that "communication across languages involves more than just a literal transfer of information" (Temple and Edwards, 2002, p.2). Translation is not only the technical transmission of one word to another. It is not words that are translated but meanings and concepts. That is why "the solution to many of the translator's dilemmas are not to be found in dictionaries, but rather in an understanding of the way language is tied to local realities (*ibid.*: 3). Simon (1996) illustratively concludes that "in fact the process of meaning transfer has less to do with *finding* the cultural inscription of a term than reconstructing its value." Temple and Edwards (2002, p.6) have accentuated the "triple subjectivity" of research when three types of interactions occur: interaction between the research participant, researcher and interpreter. This three-level interaction cannot be erased but must be *made explicit*.

The analysis of gathered data can be divided into three main steps. The first step consisted of taking notes during and immediately after the interview. This was especially important for further re-consideration of the structure of the interview scenario, and for recording my reflections on what was said, how it was said, and what was observed during the interview – such as emotions, gestures, as well as artifacts, such as photos with nannies and children). The second step in the data analysis was transcription of the interview. Listening to the voices of my interviewees was important for re-evoking the atmosphere of the moment, spontaneous reactions, and many important elements which—when put on the paper—were lost. Once the interviews were transcribed, the third step began: reading the material. Repeated readings of the transcribed interviews were followed by *open coding* and simultaneous writing of the notes. Both of these activities were performed in accordance with my research questions and analytical positions. The outcome of open coding was a selective set of topics which were further elaborated. These topics were: motivations to hire/become a nanny as part of the migratory/caring biographies; negotiations of boundaries and bonding; articulation of ethnic, racial and class differences; meanings of care-giving and mothering; the role of kinship terminology in the nanny-child relationship.

The decision to study the care work relationship from three different perspectives shaped by differing social and cultural contexts was a great challenge for analysis. In my sample, I had three distinct parties with their particular standpoints, opinions, and interpretations of the relationship, and of what the other parties do. When focusing on a given topic I compared the statements of mothers, nannies, and children, and contextualized each of these statements within the interviewees' biography, tracing the origins of these statements, motivations for them, and their outcomes in the context of their self-presentation in the interviews. All this was carried out in interaction with my research objectives and the theoretical framework that channeled my analysis and writing. All this focused on the character of the relationships between mothers, children, and nannies, and how these relationships can be understood through the lens of the mutual dependency.

As an in-depth qualitative study based on a purposive sampling, this book does not claim to be generalizable. This section has outlined my research strategy as well as the limitations of my research. The analysis presented in the following pages focuses on a *particular group* of Vietnamese immigrants (first generation parents and second generation children) that employs a *specific model* of childcare, and this must be kept in mind when reading the research findings.

1.3 Plan of the Book

Chapter 2 *("We Are Here Alone": The Hiring Decision in the Struggle for Family Resettlement)* and Chapter 3 *("We Need Each Other": Childcare as a Paid and Fulfilling Activity)* explain the recruitment decisions of parents and nannies. Chapter 2 focuses on what motivates Vietnamese families to recruit Czech nannies, while Chapter 3 analyzes why some Czech women become nannies in Vietnamese families. These chapters provide readers with the essential first step for understanding the nature of emerging relationships between nannies, mothers, and children. In Chapter 2 I argue that the hiring decision is an inherent part of family re-settlement, where parents are confronted with their own cultural roots and ideas about care-giving/mothering, which clash with the structural care arrangements defined in Czech family policy. Upon leaving Vietnam, families left older family generations behind, and have had to construct new forms of intergenerational solidarity in the new country. The main conclusion here is that a nanny *fulfils the ideal of relatives in family life*, and that she supplants the mother and supplements the grandmother. Chapter 3 shows how the needs of immigrant Vietnamese families are met by employing Czech women as nannies. The nannies, almost exclusively dependent on the welfare state (unemployed or retired), are a perfect match for the Vietnamese family. For different reasons, these women welcome the extra money paid care brings to their household; however, the most important reasons for taking on childcare responsibilities comes from the Czech women's individual life biographies. The women had subjective motivations for becoming nannies, and utilized care work to construct their gendered caring biographies according to the local gender norms and their individual social preferences (e.g. the nannies' kinship and intergenerational relations). Revealing the non-economic side of their motivations, this chapter allows us to overcome the bipolar framework of childcare/domestic work, which assumes that nannies are poor immigrant women, who work for well-off native women. In addition, it opens space for addressing the issue of gendered biographies as a main source of care-giving work, rather than focusing on care-giving as solely a breadwinning activity.

Chapter 4 *("Everything for Us but Nothing with Us": Meaning of Motherhood, Delegation of Care Work and its Consequences)* looks at how the various resources for realizing motherhood and ideas and ideals about motherhood clash in the nanny-mother relationship, and how the images of good motherhood are mutually constructed. At the same time, the delegation of motherhood is analyzed from the point of view of the children, focusing on how they comprehend the delegation of care, and how this delegation impacts their understanding of inter-generational ties and the family. This chapter shows that the Vietnamese work ethic is not based on the ideas of self-realization (as in western parts of Europe), but rather on saving money for the future of their children. The family is primarily an economic unit meant to support social upward mobility for the next generations. It is more important for mothers to work and earn money for the future of their children than to be socially and emotionally present in their children's everyday lives. Passing the daily mothering work on to the nannies, the mothers do their mothering in the labour market, by providing for children financially and emotionally, by proxy, through the nannies. How do the nannies and children perceive such definition of motherhood? This question is answered in Chapter 4, and leads us to consider the broader implication of delegated motherhood in the lives of first and second immigrants and their integration.

Chapter 5 *("From Nanny to Granny": Caring as Kinning)* and Chapter 6 (*"Europe is My Brain, Asia is My Heart": GrandMotherland and Kinning as Home-Bonding*) address the link between care-giving, kinning and home-bonding. The case of migrant children having native nannies take care of them reveals the essential role of care-giving when defined in terms of relationships: the link between care-giving and kinning (Chapter 5), as well as the link between kinning and home-bonding (Chapter 6). Chapter 5 traces the process of kinning in which the second generation Vietnamese children are subjectified into grandchildren and nannies into grandmothers. I borrow the concept of kinning from Howell (2003) to illuminate the daily negotiations of being/becoming a member of a family and the diverse activities during which the children are assigned their role as grandchildren and nannies are assigned their role as the children's grandmothers. Consequently, Chapter 6 focuses on the role of kinning and kinship ties in accounts of belonging to homeland. This chapter challenges the primordial definitions of belonging (when illuminating how home-bonds are thought of as attained, developed, and performed) and demonstrates its endurance (when the homeland is naturalized and imagined through the symbolism of blood and genes). These chapters track the similarities between accounts of kinship and accounts of belonging, and cover the broad issue of establishing and maintaining kinship ties both through the everyday practice of care, and through the feeling of belonging to a genealogy. The main contribution of these chapters lies in its stress on the formative role of caring in establishing a sense of kinship as well as sense of belonging to a new national homeland. I address here the pervasive ambivalence between biogenetic and social relatedness in the children's and nannies' perception of selfhood, and the children's and nannies' position in the two, complex frames of reference for the children's and nannies' identity and belonging—kinship and national homeland.

And finally, in Chapter 7, I conclude by considering the broader theoretical implications of my work. Returning to the initial research questions, this chapter distinguishes several layers of mutual dependencies, and shows what we can learn from the particular experience of immigrant Vietnamese families hiring native nannies in the Czech Republic.

With its stress on mutuality in care work, this book illuminates the new forms of interpersonal, interethnic, and intergenerational relationships emerging in the twenty-first century. It stresses the mechanisms and processes in which the kinship ties are negotiated and reproduced. Therefore, it also contributes to general sociological theories on childhood, motherhood, kinship, relatedness, homeland belonging, etc. The framework adopted in this book can be useful both for mainstream research on care workers and family relations (as it is not limited to immigrant families with nannies) and for research on the second generation immigrant childhood.

* * *

This book shows how paid care-giving is contextualized in terms of various relationships between the three types of actors: employer and employee, care-giver and care-receiver, and mother-child. All of these ties are based on ontologically different principles and each of them operates as a piece of a puzzle, which is meaningful only in relation to each other. This book considers care-giving to be a formative activity that establishes ties between the concerned actors, whose subjectivities are mutually shaped in the daily practice of care-giving. The ties between nannies and mothers are based on the logic of employment (economic mutual dependency), and reflect the disagreements and tensions about what good motherhood is in relation to gendered subjectivities (mutual dependency in motherhood/womanhood definition). The ties between children and mothers are based on biological relations, but must be performed and reaffirmed in the daily practice of caring. The mother becomes a mother when she mothers/cares for her child, while the child becomes the mother's child when he/she receives care from her. And finally, ties between nannies and children are based on the mutual exchange of emotions and everyday care-giving (mutual emotional dependency), both of which lead to the establishment of kinship ties. The nannies become grandmothers and children become grandchildren (intergeneration mutual dependency and in care-giving and care-receiving as the formative aspect of family relationships).

Chapter 2
"We Are Here Alone": The Hiring Decision in the Struggle for Family Resettlement[1]

> Here we must work much more than we would in Vietnam. There I would have my family who would help me. But here I do not have anybody like that.
>
> Ms. Ho, mother of two children—Bao and Thuy

Hello, my name is Thuy Tran. I am 8 years old and after the holidays, I will go to the third grade of primary school. I have an older brother. His name is Boa Tran and he is 12 years old. I was born in the Czech Republic, here in a town close to the border with Poland. When I grow up, I want to be a doctor. I know I have to learn a lot to become one so I do my best at school. I like playing piano and I am very good at gymnastics, skiing and ice skating.

My mum's name is Ho. She was not born in the Czech Republic like me and my brother. She was born in Vietnam and came here in 1997. She did not want to leave Vietnam because she had many friends and relatives there and a very good job, but my father was already here and she wanted to be with him so she moved. It was very difficult for her to leave all my grandparents and aunts and uncles behind. She says that when she came, everything was new for her and she felt that people in the Czech Republic were not as open as they probably are in France or Australia. Today it is more than 14 years since she came here to the Czech Republic and she does not have many Czech friends (I have many more), she misses her family. On the other hand, she has many Vietnamese friends here and they are very nice and supportive. I am sure they would help us with all our problems. My mum says that the Czech Republic is her second home. I think it is because of me and my brother. My parents do not want to stay here forever. We know that when my mum gets old and me and Boa are adults and educated, she wants to return to her home country. Since 1997 she has visited Vietnam five times and she was very sad that she cannot stay there. I think it was too painful for her to come back to the Czech Republic. But I do not speak Vietnamese at all so we cannot move there. As both my mum and my dad say, they are here because of us, so now they have to stay until we are independent from them. Meanwhile, they can call up our relatives or go there for a visit.

---

1 An earlier version of this chapter was published under the title Vietnamese Immigrants in the Czech Republic: Hiring a Czech Nanny as a Post-Migratory Family Settlement Strategy (Souralová, 2014a).

When my mum came to the Czech Republic, she became an entrepreneur. Both my parents have been entrepreneurs from the beginning. We have a shop with clothes—T-shirts, trousers, even socks and so on. It takes a lot of their time to be there and sell all these colourful things. That is why my mum could not stay at home with me when I was a little baby. When Boa was 10 months old, she also had to return to work from parental leave. He had five nannies that took care of him. Then I was born and the situation was even worse, so my mum had to return to work when I was only 2 months old. I know she wanted to stay home with us longer, but my dad's income was not enough for all of us. However, I was lucky because my parents found me my nanny. They asked some friends of theirs whether they did not know of some nice, kind woman, and that is how I met my nanny. Now I have had her for eight years and I like her very much. My mum knows that she can rely on her and that I am safe with her. These days I also spend more time with her because my parents had to move their business to Slovakia. They said it is because of the economic crisis. They work there and come to see me and my brother only on Sundays. That is why I live with my nanny now.

* * *

Many studies of childcare and domestic work suggest that nannies are usually immigrants working in middle-class professional families (for a critique see Macdonald, 2010). It seems that such a pattern of relationships begs the very basic question of why a woman recruits another woman—coming from different cultural, social, and geographic context—to take care of her child. It also begs the question of why the one woman would want to be hired as a nanny and work for the other woman? It is assumed that the motivations on both sides are the result of the structural position of these women. It is further assumed that women seeking childcare are employed in managerial and professional positions, in a labour market segment that is based on the model of an unencumbered male worker who is free of family responsibilities and able to put in extensive working hours (Macdonald, 2010). On the other side of the relationship, the *immigrant* women's motivations to become nannies are typically understood within an economic framework, in which these women generally work as nannies because they must work and earn money. Domestic work, as Ayse Akalin (2008, p.103) argues, "is a significantly lucrative kind of work for migrants whose main motivation is to make and save as much money as they can for their needs at home." Both arguments fit perfectly into the international scholarship on domestic work, in which hiring a nanny is understood as a means to reconcile family and work life and solve public problems (the lack of child care facilities) with private solutions (informally hiring a nanny).

In the following two chapters an analysis of the motivations for hiring and becoming a nanny are presented. I explore the interplay of motivations for the demand and supply of paid child care in the context of post-migratory lives on the one hand, and care biographies on the other. To capture the dynamic interplay of the incentives on both sides, I trace the decisions to hire/become a nanny as the resolution of a mutual need, which leads to the emergence of mutual dependency in the relationship. I argue that such an approach is a useful tool for understanding the motivations because: firstly, it allows us to overcome the bipolar framework of child care/domestic work that suggests an activity performed by poor women for rich women. And secondly, it gives us a chance to comprehend the complementary mutuality of the relationship, which are two of the essential aspects of paid child care in this case study that make the relationship sustainable.

In Chapter 2 I aim to answer the basic question: Why do Vietnamese families hire nannies to look after their children? After a brief overview on Vietnamese immigration to the Czech Republic, I will deal with the dual questions of why Vietnamese families in my sample hire *nannies*, and why Vietnamese families in my sample hire *Czech* nannies, specifically. I argue that the answers cannot be found if we regard the recruitment of nannies merely as the only way to reconcile work and family life as necessary after the gender revolution and the feminization of the work force. Instead the motivations are far more complex, and must be interpreted in the context of post-migratory redefinition of family life and generational relationship negotiations. The two key words around which the whole chapter turns are, thus, *(post-migratory) settlement* and *family (kinship) life*. Therefore I will start with a brief history of Vietnamese immigration to the Czech Republic/Czechoslovakia, which created the macro-structural context of the family settlement, "a series of microprocesses related to household and family establishment" (Hondagneu-Sotelo, 1994, p.18). I then turn to understanding the hiring decisions as one of these microprocesses, and stress its role in "replanting" the uprooted families.

2.1 (Temporal) Migration and (Imagined) Return

In the interviews, when asking interviewees about their or their parents' migration experience, I heard a number of different stories. A very common pattern experienced by many of the families in the study was described in the interview with Thi, a 22-year-old university student, who was born in Vietnam and came to the Czech Republic at the age of three: "My dad studied here in the 1980s, then he came back to Vietnam and in the 1990s the big boom of Vietnamese markets started so he decided to return here, at that time it was Czechoslovakia. And me and my mum, we joined him in 1994 thanks to family reunification." These four lines of Thi's story sum up the basic experience of Vietnamese migration to the Czech Republic.

The experience of migration to this country differs fundamentally from that of Vietnamese migrants to capitalist countries beginning in the 1970s. The geopolitical situation at that time produced two parallel streams of migration from Vietnam corresponding to the two sides of the Cold War. The turning point in Vietnamese migration to the Czech Republic and the countries of Central and Eastern Europe was 1989, when the Soviet bloc fell apart and the nature of migration to what was then still Czechoslovakia changed completely. Migration from Vietnam was thus shaped by two radically differing migration regimes: before 1989 in the context of state socialism it was a strictly state-managed migration between two socialist countries with closed borders (personified by Thi's father who studied in socialist Czechoslovakia); after 1989 it became a classic labour migration shaped by privatization and marketization (which Thi describes as "the Vietnamese outdoor market boom"; see Baláž and Williams, 2007; Brouček, 2003). As Baláž and Williams (2007, p.43) remark, and as we can see from Thi's statement, the two phases were not autonomous or disconnected from one another; instead "the pathway(s) of the first phase migrants intersected with and informed pathway of the second phase—especially via social network and migrant-host community relationships—shaping opportunities and constraints for both groups." In the next part I briefly sum up the routes and roots of Vietnamese migration to the CR, and its consequences for the current situation of Vietnamese migrants in Czech society, as well as for the Czech nannies they hire.

The origins of Thi's father's opportunity to come to come Czechoslovakia as a student can be found in the mid-1950s. In 1956 the first international agreement enabled the arrival of individuals and 100 children afflicted by war (Brouček, 2003). At the same time several bilateral agreements were signed on economic-cultural cooperation (1955), scientific-technological cooperation (1956), and cultural cooperation (1957). These agreements allowed students from Vietnam to come in the 1960s. After spending one year in Czech language school, they were enrolled in study programs chosen by the Vietnamese, the majority of them in technical programs. A few of them started to study Czech language and literature or puppet-acting (Martínková, 2006). However, the most important breaking point was the year 1973, when Vietnam displayed increased interest in communication with Czechoslovakia, and asked for the admission into the Czech labour force in various occupations—both for training and for employment. Economic and political cooperation increased after Vietnam's reunification in 1975, and over the two following years when the "Agreements on Mutual Assistance" were signed between Vietnam and several CEE states (Williams and Baláž, 2005). In 1978 Vietnam became a member of the Council for Mutual Economic Assistance, and its "integration into the Soviet block was completed" (Williams and Baláž, 2005, p.536).

The number of Vietnamese immigrants coming on the basis of agreements reached its peak between 1980 and 1983, when 30 000 students, apprentices, and young workers from Vietnam lived in the former Czechoslovakia (Brouček, 2003). The task of these immigrants (in large part men), whose arrival to CEE countries was an expression of socialist solidarity, was simple: learn from a more developed "brother country," develop human capital, and help Vietnam to recover after years of war (Williams and Baláž, 2005). At the beginning their stay was limited to four or seven years, and in the 1980s the workers were urged to return to their homeland to fulfil this mission. A new bilateral agreement was reached to decrease the number of the Vietnamese in CEE, and two thirds of the immigrants went back to Vietnam—among them Thi's father. To sum up with Williams and Baláž (2005, p.546), Vietnamese immigration to Central Eastern European countries is to be understood "in the context of how cold war geopolitics and the notion of 'global brotherhood' (with gender connotations) structured human mobility."

The fall of communism in 1989 naturally meant the termination of agreements, and gave rise to a new stage in Vietnamese migration to Czechoslovakia. It also opened new work possibilities for those Vietnamese who stayed in the host country, as the pressure to return to Vietnam was eased (Brouček, 2003). There were generally two possibilities for those who did not return to Vietnam: either they could emigrate to Western countries (as their previous stay in Europe made possible), or they could stay in Czechoslovakia and legalize their residence there (Brouček, 2003). One of the easiest means of legalization was to apply for a business license, which was also the best solution *vis-à-vis* the new labour market situation and the disappearance of the jobs that Vietnamese workers held before 1989 (Hofírek and Nekorjak, 2009). Now a new chapter of Vietnamese immigration to the Czechoslovakia began to be written and migration slowly became a standard economic labour migration, and since the beginning of the 1990s, Vietnamese returnees from the era of socialist cooperation, their relatives, and friends have come to make use of the new opportunity to carry on business and become part of the immigrant economy of entrepreneurs (see below). Thi's father, who responded to (as Thi put it) the "big boom of Vietnamese markets," was one of them. The number of immigrants started increasing also thanks to family reunification, which allowed Thi, for example, to come to the Czech Republic.

Today Vietnamese immigrants are the third largest group in the Czech Republic after Ukrainians and Slovaks. Approximately 60 thousand Vietnamese people live here, which is around 15 percent of the entire immigrant population, and 0.6 percent of the whole population. The historical specificity of managed migration from Vietnam to CEE and the continuing migration after the fall of communism in 1989 has a strong impact on the character of the Vietnamese diaspora in the CEE up to this day (Williams and Baláž, 2005). Two features of the Vietnamese diaspora in the Czech Republic are crucial for this book. First is the demographic structure of the Vietnamese population. Compared to other groups of immigrants, the demographic structure of the Vietnamese immigrant population is progressive, with a high percentage of women and children. According to the Czech Statistical Office, in 2005, 21 percent of the Vietnamese population were children 0–14 years old (in the Czech population it was 15 percent) and 78 percent of the population are of working age (15–64), with only 1 percent being older than 65 years old.

Second, the employment structure of the Vietnamese population is characterized by high occupational concentration. A large proportion of Vietnamese immigrants are entrepreneurs in wholesaling and retailing, i.e. owners of small shops and/or open-air markets (Williams and Baláž, 2005; 2007). Self-employment is thus the crucial aspect of their working life in the Czech Republic. In 2009, around 88,000 (63,000 men and 25,000 women) foreigners in the Czech Republic held a valid trade license; of these some 36,000 were Vietnamese (25,000 men and 11,000 women). As mentioned above, self-employment became a strategy for legalizing one's residence (Hofírek and Nekorjak, 2009). Vietnamese entrepreneurs mobilized their "human capital, ethnic networks and family/community solidarity" and developed trading activities that filled a particular market gap in the economy. Becoming petty traders, Vietnamese immigrants "were the early winners in the globalization of the Slovak [and Czech] economy after 1989" (Williams and Baláž, 2005, p.540). However, shortly before the economic crisis in 2008, competition from international hypermarkets and stores was slowly turning these Vietnamese businesspeople into losers in the new globalized economy (*ibid.*). Some immigrant entrepreneurs began re-orienting their businesses in new directions, such as convenience stores, nail studios, etc. However, the emphasis on petty trading still prevails, and this is very much echoed in the interviews.[2]

Labour-oriented migration figures in the accounts as the chance to give children a better life. Experiences with war and poverty very often become an issue during interviews with children; the collective memory of suffering is conveyed to them and rhetorically used as an argument to justify the migration project. A recurring argument in the account is that the only goal of migration for the first generation is to ensure a better future for their children. As such, when giving meaning to the migratory experience, interviewees and/or their parents talk about the temporary nature of this migration, and their plan to return to the homeland. Lien, an 18-year old girl born in a Czech town close to the Czech-German border, told me during the interview that she is very much aware of the fact that her parents are only in the Czech Republic because of her and her brother.

> Our parents want to return to Vietnam, it is one hundred percent. My mum says that when I have my own family, my own background, my own husband and maybe also children, then she will say to herself 'my daughter has her own life.' And when she can say this, she will leave because she has already accomplished her mission here and she has nothing else to do here in the Czech Republic. My parents do not have any friends here, no family, the people around them are only the Vietnamese who only work, they are here for their kids to have the best education, you know, European education, European habits, European friends and generally better standards. That is why they toil from morning to evening because of their kids.

This story, told by many interviewees, expresses two important issues in the lives of Vietnamese immigrants. First is the temporary nature of the parents' stay in the host country, the goal of which is to build satisfactory conditions for their children's life, and then to leave. This goes against the general interpretation of

2 For instance, Ms. Ho (introduced at the beginning of this chapter) and her husband solved the decline of their clothing store by moving their shop 170 kilometers from the place where they lived with their children, to Slovakia, and not by trying to change their jobs.

a progressive demographic structure of an immigrant group, which follows this logic: if the immigrants start families in the host country, it is an indicator of their attempt to assimilate and stay there. However, in my data, the *idea of return* (meaning a plan and a *longing* to return home to Vietnam) was a strong part of the accounts. Second, such temporality permeates the everyday life of Vietnamese parents who, like Lien's, lack social networks, and most of their friends share their geographical origin. This leads not only to the general picture of Vietnamese immigrants as a closed community in the eyes of the majority, but above all, to difficulty on the part of Vietnamese immigrants' in developing a relationship to the host country, social contacts, or language competencies.

2.2 Post-Migratory Family Challenges and Patterns

Vietnamese families hiring Czech nannies find themselves in the awkward position of attempting to reconstruct family life—firstly, after arrival in the host country, and secondly, after a nanny enters the family/household and takes over childcare responsibilities. While Chapter 5 deals with the negotiation of kinship ties when a nanny enters the arena of care work, here I analyze delegated child care as a result of post-migratory changes in family life. Immigrant family life has been the subject of a number of studies that have shown how life in the new country leads immigrants to reconcile their old and new ideas about family life which is marked by conflicting processes of change and struggles for continuity (Kibria, 1993; Foner, 1997; Hondagneu-Sotelo, 1994). On a general level Nancy Foner (1997, p.962) writes that

> The cultural understandings, meanings, and symbols that immigrants bring with them from their home societies are also critical in understanding immigrant family life. Obviously, immigrants do not reproduce exactly their old cultural patterns when they move to a new land; but these patterns continue to have a powerful influence in shaping family values and norms as well as actual patterns of behaviour that develop in the new setting.

My main source of inspiration for understanding why Vietnamese immigrants in the Czech Republic hire nannies is the work of Nazli Kibria, from 1993. In her study of Vietnamese immigrants in the USA—suitably entitled "Family Tightrope"—, the author follows the generational and gender relations of families resettling in the United States. She describes how the new economic and social context in which these families find themselves produces complicated family situations (the family tightrope) balancing between the Vietnamese and American cultures, and leads to complicated negotiations over the meaning of the family, the household, and relationships within it. She shows, *inter alia*, that the way immigrant families live under the new structural conditions, and the way they respond to these conditions, is affected by the "cultural baggage, or experience and understanding about the world, that they bring with them to the new society" (Kibria, 1993, p.22). Here I will argue that the recruitment of nannies in Vietnamese families is part of the complex process of resettling the family, balancing between the home and host countries, between then and now, and negotiating a new family life, including ways of caring for children in the new country. I focus here on three main turning points brought about by the arrival in a new country:

1. the change in the work environment, which raises the question of *how to combine work and family life*;
2. a transnational balancing between two cultural worlds, which leads to a *rethinking and combining of family models from the home and host countries*; and
3. displacement from the social network, which presents the dilemma of *how to deal with the new family situation without the support of the extended family*. The combined effect of these three factors is a new constellation of relationships within the family, which results in the decision to hire a Czech nanny.

2.2.1 New Work Life: "We Are Foreigners here so We Have to Work More"

I was often told by interviewees that there is only one *real* reason why they recruit nannies: parents have to work; they cannot survive in the host country on one salary, and the woman must return to work (either to help her husband in his shop or to run her own) as soon as possible. Vietnamese families thus present one of the most common scenarios for those seeking childcare services: Dual-earner families, where both parents are working outside the home demand care work. In the initial phase of research in the spring of 2010, I received a contact for Ms. Veselá (born Nguyen)—a woman from Vietnam that came to the former Czechoslovakia before 1989, married a Czech, and works at present as a translator. When I requested an interview with her, she agreed immediately, and gave me the following instructions: "Let's meet tomorrow and I will take you somewhere where you'll understand why the Vietnamese do this." The next day Ms. Veselá picked me up at the agreed upon place and took me to Brno's biggest outdoor market. We walked among the stands that sell clothing and food, all operated by Vietnamese people of all ages and family status. We came to a small fast-food place, where we ordered strong Vietnamese coffee. As we were drinking our coffee, Ms. Veselá told me to look around carefully, and then asked, "Now you understand it all, don't you?" At that point I realized that Vietnamese families' commitment to their work should be understood as the main reason why they hire women to watch their children. In case I had any doubts, Ms. Veselá explained in detail:

> Generally, the Vietnamese are taught that people of productive age must work, and being on maternity leave is not work. Everybody must work; parents, grandparents, and older children and kids have all done it since childhood. Here

> [in the Czech Republic] they have their shops, they are entrepreneurs, so that they do not want or they cannot close the shop. For them, when the shop is closed, the goods are not sold, there is no profit, and the clients do not come again. It is impossible to close the shop for a week or two and go for a holiday with the family. They are able to pay an education for their kids; they send them to England for three weeks to learn English, which is very expensive. They are able to pay for that; but to close the shop and go for holiday with kids, that is a waste of time, they would say.

Many of my other interviewees cited work commitments as the most important reason for seeking a nanny. Thus my understanding of the role of the nanny in the lives of Vietnamese immigrants began with understanding their work life, which merges around three common tensions that are often mentioned in interviews with children and mothers.

First is the tension between working in Vietnam and working in the Czech Republic. It would be misleading to consider the creation of a dual-earner household as a function only of geographical mobility and the desire to better one's life in the host country. When Ms. Veselá says that the Vietnamese learn that everybody of productive age must work, she is making a statement repeated in many interviews. The dual-earner household is already in place in Vietnam before coming to the Czech Republic. However, for both men and women work life radically changes after crossing borders. In particular, there are qualitative changes in work biographies when immigrants shift from their previous professions (skilled or unskilled), and become entrepreneurs in the immigrant economy. This was also the case for those immigrants who—like Thi's father—came to Czechoslovakia before 1989 as students and graduated from university. For them, being part of the immigrant economy means working in low-skill jobs for which they are often overqualified.

In addition, the new occupational position requires quantitative changes in work life, and leads to its intensification at the expense of private life, as the logic "close the shop, you will earn nothing" shapes the meaning of labour, especially in a period of economic crisis. The interviewees experience what Wall and José (2004) called pressures *to* work—as the migration project aims at maximizing income—and pressures *from* work, such as atypical or long hours and the pressure not to miss work. Because they struggled to come to a new country, and had to compete in a very competitive segment of economy, Vietnamese immigrant women were aware of the fragility of their position. Six months after giving birth to her daughter, Ms. Pham faced the dilemma of whether to hire a shop assistant or a nanny. At the time, her husband had found a place for a new shop where she could sell clothes, and she had to make a quick decision. So she decided to hire a nanny for her 7-month-old daughter.

A second tension is closely linked to the first one, and involves that of being Vietnamese working in the Czech Republic. Besides stating that "if I were in Vietnam, I would work less," the interviewees also say that "if I were Czech, I would work less." If the goal of migration is to ensure a better future for one's children, work is the means to achieve this end. Vietnamese parents must work more than Czech parents because Vietnamese children enter society with the stigma of being foreigners. As Chapter 4 will show, parents' intensive incorporation into the labour market and self-sacrifice in breadwinning activity are essential part of their definition of "good parenthood." Working hard and creating dual-earner households is not a form of self-realization of one's ambitions, but rather responsible performance of one's of one's parental role.

A third tension—and the one most evident in my interviews—is that of balancing work and family life in the Czech Republic. Many research studies have reported that Vietnamese immigrant families experience a conflict between work and childcare, and feel they "have so much to do that they feel they have a hard time managing everyday life" (Forsberg, 2009, p.162). Ms. Veselá's statement—which was very much echoed in the interviews with children— demonstrates that for Vietnamese immigrants, *everyday* life is *work* life. For sacrificing their private lives to earn money, Vietnamese parents are both admired and chastised by their children. The conflict arises when parents employ strategies for reconciling family and work life learned in Vietnam, in the Czech Republic. These efforts to harmonize home and work life are understood and experienced differently by parents and by children. For the parents the Czech Republic is a place where one *works*, while for the children it is a place where one *lives and settles.* Parents are in the Czech Republic *because of* their kids but are not truly *with* their kids there. The parents' lack of a private life becomes a big issue for the second generation, who experience misunderstandings with parents (both linguistic and human) and a confused sense of belonging).

All the children recognize that their parents' are sacrificing their personal life for them (the children), and they greatly admire their parents for being able to work so much. Nevertheless, lack of time spent together as a family was a sore issue for all my child interviewees. When I met Thi, and we talked about life, she said with sadness in her voice that her parents worked so much that they did not have time either for themselves or for her. "I know they do it for me, but I would prefer if they took one day off and made a trip with me," she sighed. Later during our talk she expressed regret about her parents' life: "My parents are satisfied in the Czech Republic, they are used to the conditions here and they kind of like it here. Nevertheless, it is not their home because since they have been here, it is 20 years now, and they only work and do not have any fun, which is a pity."

2.2.2 (Transnational) Child Care Models Balancing: "It is Normal in Vietnam"

All the Vietnamese families are part of what Peggy Levitt and Nina Glick Schiller (2004) called a transnational social field. Watching Vietnamese television, calling and chatting with friends and relatives back in Vietnam, remittances sent to the homeland, home visits and the idea of return, all shape their transnational lives. Vietnamese parents consequently have more frames of reference at their disposal, and this equips them with multiple sources of ideas about what the family is and how care is performed. In other words, child care is ideologically organized around the model from Vietnam ("how we would have done it if we had been in Vietnam," "how we did it when we were still in Vietnam," "how our parents did it," "how our sisters and brothers do it"), but it is geographically bounded by the Czech Republic where the care is performed.

Contrasting childcare strategies in Vietnam and the Czech Republic, Vietnamese mothers highlighted the radical difference between maternal leave policies and child care facilities in the two countries. In Vietnam, the total time for paid maternal leave varies from four months (for normal types of employment); five months (for employment in dangerous environments or difficult shifts, such as policewomen or soldiers) to six months (if a woman is disabled). Women are paid 100 percent of their salary during these four months; thereafter, employees can request unpaid maternal leave (Nguyen, 2012, p.7). As my interviewees state, only rich families can afford unpaid maternal leave because, as argued above, two salaries are a necessity, especially in poorer regions. Maternal leave arrangements thus create the demand for both formal and informal childcare facilities. Formal childcare is provided in public and private schools and centers: nursery schools (for children aged 3 months–3 years), kindergarten (3–5 years) and pre-primary schools (5–6 years). Nevertheless, despite this net of institutions, most families with children under 3 years old rely on informal childcare (Nguyen, 2012). To my question of how Vietnamese parents would have managed the child care if they had stayed in Vietnam, almost all the interviewees answered that the mother returning to the workplace would be replaced by the grandmother, or in richer families, by private nannies or maids.

Such experiences (whether personal or generalized) and ideas about childcare models are challenged in the host country, where current childcare and general family policies are marked by the reintroduction of the traditional "familization" regime (Sirovátka and Saxonberg, 2006; Lister, *et al.* 2007). As Tomáš Sirovátka and Steven Saxonberg (2006, p.185) argue in their analysis of post-1989 family policies, "when the communist walls came tumbling down, Central European women found themselves in a historically unique situation. On the one hand, they experienced the highest employment levels in the entire world, with only the Scandinavian social democratic countries coming close. On the other hand, in contrast to the Scandinavian countries, little discussion arose about the need for men to share in household and child-rearing chores. As a result, the household remained strictly the domain of the woman." It is important to say that among these "women in a historically unique situation" were also nannies currently working for Vietnamese families. However, Vietnamese parents arriving in the Czech Republic in early 1990s witnessed a radical shift in family policies, which meant a promotion of state support for women to stay at home with children.

What happened? Sirovátka and Saxonberg analyze three key areas that "influence the ability for women and men to balance work and family: childcare leave schemes, access to daycare and labor market policies" (Sirovátka and

Saxonberg, 2006, p.186). Here I will briefly mention the first and second areas, as they are crucial for my interviewees. In the Czech Republic (as well as in other CEE countries), there are two kinds of paid family leave. First is maternity leave benefits, which have not changed since the fall of communism, and are still available for 28 weeks, with a replacement rate of 69 percent in the Czech Republic (Sirovátka and Saxonberg, 2006). Parental leave is available for as long as four years, and it is up to the parents (most often the mother) to choose the length and hence the level of the replacement rate. The amount of money for four years is 220,000 CZK. This means that a parent can draw the money for 19 months (a monthly amount of almost 12, 000) up to 45 months (at around 5,100 a month). The Vietnamese mothers I interviewed regarded parental leave as "too long" and for them inappropriate. Although they agreed that they would *surely* like to stay home longer with children, four years (the maximum parental leave) meant for them an unimaginable break in their working life.

The explicit re-familization policy, "which promotes separate gender roles for men and women, since few men will be willing to utilize their right to parental leave under these conditions" (*ibid.*, p.189) is further confirmed by the reduction of state aid for nursery schools for children 0–3 years old. This reduction was accompanied by an attack on the mythologies regarding collective daycare for children under 3. Nursery schools were declared to be a "communist invention" (Hašková and Dudová, 2010), and collective care for 0–3 aged children "unhealthy" and/or "unnecessary" (Hašková and Saxonberg, 2012). Table 2.1 illustrates how the network of nursery schools has been reduced.

Table 2.1 Numbers of nursery schools and numbers of placed children

	1990	1991	1995	1998	2001	2004	2007	2011
Establishments	1043	486	207	79	59	58	47	45
Places	39829	-	7574	2191	1717	1708	1495	1425

Note: by December 31 of each year.
Source: Institute of Health Information and Statistics of the Czech Republic.

However, the lack of nursery schools is not the only factor that shapes Vietnamese parents' childcare decisions. Even in districts where childcare facilities are available, the lack of flexibility creates an important barrier. Generally nursery schools are open until 5 pm, which is not sufficient for the parents who work until 8 or 9 pm (in urban areas). Even if they managed to place the children in nursery schools, parents would need someone to pick them up and stay with them until they came from work. It seems, therefore, that existing daycare arrangements are not convenient for (Vietnamese) working parents.

To sum up, Vietnamese parents experience big differences between childcare models in Vietnam and in the Czech Republic. In their effort to follow the Vietnamese model (returning to work after four months' maternal leave), Vietnamese parents face a radically different situation in the Czech Republic. First, the relatively long paid family leave and negative mythologies regarding collective childcare shape the discourse of what Ann Oakley (1974) called the "myth of motherhood," and Sharon Hays labelled the ideology of intensive mothering (1996) in the USA. Re-familization policies in the Czech Republic strengthened the ideology of a gendered division of reproductive labour, and created the model of the permanent, individual caregiver (read: mother). The issue of how these general meanings of motherhood/childcare are accomplished in biographies of nannies and mothers will be broadly discussed in Chapter 4. Second, childcare facilities that provide important institutional support in Vietnam are in the Czech Republic, either far away, full, or unusable because of early closing hours. If the childcare facilities were unavailable in Vietnam, Vietnamese parents would delegate the childcare to their kin—usually grandmothers. How can this very common option in Vietnam be employed in the Czech Republic?

3.2.3 Dislocation from Kinship Networks: "We Do not Have Anybody here"

Nguyet, a 20-year-old university student, came to the Czech Republic when she was 4 years old. Before they moved to the Czech Republic, Nguyet's mother went back to work immediately after a four-month maternity leave. Four-month-old Nguyet was taken care of by her grandmother, her mother's mother. When the family moved to the CR, her mother again had to take a job, and needed to find a *substitute for her mother* who had looked after Nguyet in Vietnam. And so she found her daughter a nanny. As is apparent in this example, the Czech nanny in the Vietnamese family supplements the mother and supplants the grand-mother (Nelson, 1990).

The role of kinship relations in delegated care has been described in a few studies (such as Uttal, 1999), some of which are devoted to the role of social/kinship relations in the post-migration harmonization of employment and family life (Moon, 2003). The absence of a network of relatives impacts many areas of post-migration life. In my interviewees' accounts, it is often spoken of in terms of a lack of economic and emotional support. Nevertheless, it is precisely the question of taking care of children—in view of the important role played in childcare by grandparents in Vietnam—that is a major point of friction, and where the loss of kinship networks is most keenly felt. For Nguyet's mother, as for other interviewees, the hiring of a nanny represents an alternative strategy simulating the previous model of childcare, in which the task is delegated to grandparents. To the question of "How would you deal with looking after the children if you were in Vietnam?" the majority answered clearly that the grandmother would take over for the mother when the latter had return to work. As one of the nannies tellingly put it, "They don't have their grandmothers here, so they have to find some." Nevertheless, why do they find *Czech* nannies?

2.3 Czech Nannies: Available and at Hand

So far my argument has aimed at explaining why some Vietnamese families hire some nannies. I have attempted to show what gap the nannies fill in the lives of cared-for children and their parents. Having explained why Vietnamese families recruit nannies, I will now turn to the question of why Vietnamese families recruit *Czech* nannies.

In the Vietnamese community, having a Czech nanny is becoming the post-migration norm. While according to Hana Hašková only 1–2 percent of Czech families make use of individual private paid childcare (Hašková, 2008), my interviewees report that the number of Vietnamese families seeking nannies for their children is around 80–95 percent. Most of them add that this is a "common," "normal," or "matter-of-fact" thing. Following the parents' logic of providing children with a better future, I assumed that one of the main incentives for recruiting *Czech* nannies was the nanny's potential role as a teacher of the Czech language and norms for their children. In other words, I expected that the ethnicity would be a highly important factor in their decision-making. Nevertheless, my analysis of the interviews with mothers indicates that while the ethnic background of the nanny *is* an important aspect of delegated care, it is *not so* important at the moment of recruitment. In order to understand the motivations behind the decision, I argue that we must turn not only to the question of why Vietnamese families hire Czech nannies (and not Ukrainian or Vietnamese), but also why they do not hire Vietnamese nannies. These two questions will be discussed here.

To answer the first question, as to why Vietnamese families do not hire Vietnamese nannies, we must consider three interrelated factors. The first factor is the demographic composition of the Vietnamese population in the CR. As I pointed out above, only 1 percent is above 65 years of age. This has to do generally with the character of work-related migration (i.e. people of productive age are the ones who move here), and the fact that many plan to return to their home country after their productive time is finished (see above). The first answer to the question "why *not* Vietnamese nannies," is that they are simply not available; there are few Vietnamese women of non-productive age in the Czech Republic. A second factor is the nature of the immigration project; that is, the fact that Vietnamese come to the Czech Republic and live here because of work. This means that even Vietnamese immigrant women over 65 years are working and have no time to look after children. During my research I encountered only one example of a family that had grandparents in the CR. However, both of them were working, and during the week the children were taken care of by a Czech grandmother; the Vietnamese grandparents saw them only sometimes on Sunday. The last, but not least important factor is the cultural (symbolic) value of child rearing and how it is valued in relation to work within the framework of the Vietnamese community. We can find this in the attitude towards the importance of maternity leave expressed above by Ms. Veselá. For the Vietnamese "maternity leave is not work," as she emphasized during the interview; and to my question about what kind of Vietnamese women look after children, she answered "women who don't have better work than looking after some kids (…) and are incapable of doing business, so they have to do something worse that pays less." To be a nanny in the context of the Vietnamese community is not work that is sufficiently valued, either from a symbolic or financial standpoint.

To answer the question of *why Vietnamese families hire Czech nannies*, we must turn both to the nannies' biographies, which will be broadly discussed in next chapter, and which make them "available and at hand" (comparing to the Vietnamese nannies) and to the fact that these women are Czech; that is, they can teach the children some things that their Vietnamese parents cannot. All the mothers and nannies I interviewed understood childcare—no matter whether performed by mothers or nannies—not only as nurture, but above all as the transmission of social and cultural capital (Macdonald, 2010; Bourdieu, 2001). Such a conceptualization of care had two consequences for choosing between a Czech or Vietnamese nanny. When I asked my mother-interviewees whether they would prefer a Vietnamese nanny to a Czech one, they explicitly referred to the linguistic advantages of having a *Vietnamese* nanny. For instance, Ms. Duong noted: "Having a Vietnamese nanny would be the best way to teach our kids their language [Vietnamese] from early childhood. Later in kindergarten they can learn the second [Czech language]. They will be fluent in two languages and their Vietnamese will be better than if they had started later."

As the statements by Ms. Duong and others suggest, the primary reason for having a Czech nanny is not linguistic, as Vietnamese mothers are confident their children will learn Czech in any event, once they enter kindergarten. Although mothers acknowledge the role of a Czech nanny in teaching Czech, in helping with homework, and with forming social ties with members of the majority society, they are aware of the unintended consequences of their decisions—the most significant of which is their children's lack of fluency in Vietnamese. Hiring a Czech nanny is this respect a double-edged sword for Vietnamese parents. Testimonies of my mother-interviewees indicate that Vietnamese parents do not hire Czech nannies because of their supposed role as *reservoirs* of Czech language and mediators of integration. Rather, Vietnamese parents hire Czech nannies because their friends and people from the Vietnamese minority *simply do it*. In other words, Vietnamese parents did not think about having a Vietnamese nanny, but they also never thought about not having a Czech nanny.

* * *

The model in which Vietnamese families take on Czech nannies to watch their children can be interpreted in two different ways. First, it can be seen as a *strategy for reconciling working and family life*, where a dual-earner couple needs a third person to take care of the children. Second, it can be seen as a means of *fulfilling the Vietnamese ideal of relying on relatives in family life*. Two findings have led me to this conclusion: First, is the "unpacking cultural baggage" with regard to family and child care. Here we observe how Vietnamese migrants in the Czech Republic "simply do what they would do at home in Vietnam." Neither dual-earner households nor delegating child rearing to a third person are unique byproducts of Vietnamese immigration to a new country. Both phenomenon exist and have existed for a long time in Vietnam. Finding a Czech nanny does not represent a break with the traditional family model in Vietnam. Rather it is an attempt to adapt a pre-existing family model to a post-migration reality. In other words, the game does not change with immigration; both in the home and host country the mother and father both work, and the children are looked after by someone else. In the host country, the only significant change to the game is that one of the players (the grandmother) is substituted by a paid nanny. A secondary consequence of this switch of "players" is that the nanny may potentially become the children's "real grandmother." This argument will be further elaborated in Chapter 5.

Chapter 3
"We Need Each Other": Childcare as a Paid and Fulfilling Activity

> She stared at me from her baby bed, I can see it like it was today. And I stared at her and I said to myself, we need each other. I had a kind of big personal crisis those days. Well it was amazing.
>
> Ms. Dudková, nanny for Ms. Ho's daughter Thuy

Hello, my name is Thuy Tran. I am eight years old and after the holidays, I will go to the third grade of primary school. I have an older brother. His name is Boa Tran and he is 12 years old. I was born in the Czech Republic, here in a town close to the border with Poland. When I grow up, I want to be a doctor. I know I have to learn a lot to become one so I do my best at school. I like playing piano and I am very good at gymnastics, skiing and ice skating.

It was my nanny, Ms. Dudková, who taught me how to ski and ice skate. While my parents were at work, she was with me and took care of me. She is 69 years old and has two sons and three granddaughters. My nanny worked her whole life as a primary school teacher of history and Czech. She loved her job and her life was very active. She tells me a lot of stories from her former job –about pupils, trips and excursions and so on. Eight years ago, she retired. I think it was a very important event in her life. I know it because she tells about the first morning of her retirement when she woke up and opened her eyes. She says that she felt emptiness inside. And this was exactly the time when I was born. Then one of her friends asked her whether she wanted to take care of a two-month old Vietnamese girl (yes, that was me), she hesitated only until she saw me lying in my baby bed. I think she was afraid of being responsible for me because I was so little. But then she agreed of course because she had plenty of time and nothing to do. Also because her grandchildren were already grown up. I have been living with her ever since. I have my own room in her apartment with lots of toys. In the living room where we watch TV together there are a lot of pictures that I drew for my nanny and also many photos we have taken together during our trips to the mountains. I cannot imagine my parents teaching me how to ski—they do not have the time. Without my nanny, I would never ever learn this.

My nanny calls me sweetheart and I think she is very proud of me. And she has a reason for this because she taught me everything. My parents do not have enough time and now they are in Slovakia so I see them only on Sundays. So it is my nanny who visits doctors with me, talks with my teachers and helps me with everything at school. Sometimes I also meet her grandchildren, but not very often because they do not come to see her regularly. We celebrate all birthdays and Christmases. My nanny always buys me nice presents for my birthday. I love it in the summer when we barbecue together with my aunts and uncles and friends in my nanny's garden. Me and my nanny, we are together all the time and when I was smaller, people sometimes asked how come a Czech woman is taking care of a Vietnamese child. And she replied to them that I am an illegitimate child of her son (I hope he does not know about it but it is funny, isn't it?). When my nanny talks about me, she says that I am a deep source of energy for her. Recently, she started being sad and she frequently says that she is very unhappy that I am growing up so fast and she worries that I will soon tell her "bye bye" and that I will not want her anymore.

* * *

If up to now the discussion has focused on the motivations of Vietnamese families to hire nannies, it is important to shift attention to the issue of how particular women respond to the Vietnamese families' demand for nanny services, and their motivations for becoming nannies. When studying women's motivations for becoming care workers, researchers have often looked at the economic factors in decision making. The research on au pairs is an illustrative example. Authors such as Rosie Cox (2006) or Sabine Hess (2003) have indicated that the economic situation and/or post-socialist transformation in Eastern European countries are the main driving forces for young women becoming au pairs in the UK. Working as an au pair means a better income and an investment in the future. Once these women learn English, their position in the labour market in their home country improves markedly. However, many researchers challenge this exclusively economic explanation, as they argue that these women's' motivations are too complex to be understood in purely economic terms, and must be seen in terms of culture as well. For instance, Williams and Baláž (2004, p.1818) state that au pairing is "a specific lifecycle-stage experience—a rite of passage." Zuzana Búriková (2007, p.451) argues that au pairs aim through social and geographic mobility "to gain a personal freedom or power in a particular relationship and/or cultural or personal development—au pair stays are usually considered to be a lesson in growing-up and maturing."

My analysis of the motivations to become a nanny started on the assumption that economic incentives play an important but not exclusive role in women's decisions. This supposition proceeded both from the above-cited research studies, and especially from the accounts of my interviewees, who very much (I would even say *too* much) accentuated this in their description of their work. Ms. Křepelková was explicit about the economic reasons, stating that "You cannot count the hourly wage. That is simply impossible. You have less than 20 CZK.[1] And deal or no deal. But if you like doing it, then why not?" In this short quotation, the nanny refers to two essential aspects which will be discussed in this part of chapter. First is the economic side of *paid* childcare. Ms. Křepelková and other nannies agreed that taking care of Vietnamese children is an activity which can rarely be done *only* for

1 Equivalent of 1 EUR is approximately 27 CZK.

money. In 2012, the average monthly salary in the Czech Republic was just over 24,000 CZK.[2] The minimum wage in the same period was 8,000 CZK per month, which means 48 CZK per hour.[3] The average pay of the nannies in my sample was 7,000 CZK, while the most frequent pay was 6,000 CZK per month. Hence, the basic question to be answered is: Who are the women that can *afford* to take a full-time caring job, be paid a wage which is slightly below or above the minimum *monthly* salary and less than half the *hourly* salary?

The second issue to be dealt with is that of *wanting* to become a nanny and *liking* to be one. The previous chapter explored the reasons why some Vietnamese families need nannies. This chapter will explore why some Czech women need to look after Vietnamese children. I will argue that these nannies need (Vietnamese) children more than they need the money they are paid for taking care of them. (Paid) childcare holds a special meaning for nannies. It assumes a prominent place in nannies' lives because it takes up the better part of their daytime as *paid* work, and requires emotional engagement. Analyzing the motivations for becoming a nanny illuminates broader issues such as the concept of care (what is care), and the role it plays in nannies' biographies (what the care/paid childcare means to the nanny). In what follows, I will argue that the recruitment of nannies springs from the tension between economic incentives (diversification of income) and the longing for engagement, which is fulfilled by the gendered activity of caring.

3.1 Who Can Afford to be a Nanny?

Despite the diversity of biographies and incentives to become nannies, all the nannies in my sample share one common structural trait: All were dependent on the welfare state when they decided to become a nanny. The nannies particular positions in relation the welfare state, as well as their frequency in my sample, are depicted in Table 3.1.

Table 3.1 Women's position in welfare state when becoming nannies

	Nanny's Position In Welfare State					
Interviewee	Parental Leave	Unemployed	Disability Pensioner	Pensioner	Employed	Total
Nanny	1	2	3	8	1	15
Child	0	3	0	14	3	20
Mother	1	5	1	8	0	15
Total	2	10	4	30	4	50

2 Czech Statistical Office.

3 Ministry of Labor and Social Affairs.

These women's structural positions *vis-à-vis* the welfare state made them perfect candidates as nannies in Vietnamese families, which require two pre-conditions: availability and low financial demands. Both of these pre-conditions reflect the parents work and economic conditions. When it comes to availability requirement, it reflects the parents' intensive incorporation into the labour market and their work hours. The nanny must be available while parents are working and while they travel to/from their workplace. In some cases, this may amount to more than 70 hours per week (including weekends), while regular working hours in the legal labour market are 40 hours per week in the Czech Republic. Such demands consequently lead to different spatial arrangements for care-giving work, all of which variously impact on how nannies understand care work: how they perceive the boundaries between private and public; what is work and what is not; which tasks are included in and/or excluded from care-giving work (see also Hondagneu-Sotelo, 2001; Macdonald, 2010) and how ties between them and children develop. We can observe here four models of care work organization: live-in nannies, live-out nannies, live-in children and live-out children.

Table 3.2 Live-ins and live-outs

Care is performed at:	Nanny		Child	
	Lives	Takes Care	Lives	Is Cared
Child's Place	Live-In Nanny	Live-Out Nanny		
Nanny's Place			Live-In Child	Live-Out Child

Table 3.3 Live-ins and live-outs in the sample from the perspective of interviewees

Interviewees	Nanny		Child		Total
	Live-In	Live-Out	Live-In	Live-Out	
Child*	0	0	6	14	20
Nanny**	1	3	4	7	15
Mother	0	5	3	7	15
Total	1	8	13	28	50

Note: * If the child had more nannies, the nanny whom the child designated as most important is counted here. ** If the mother had more than one nanny for her child(ren), the nanny whom the mother designated as most important is counted here.

According to the place where the care is performed and whether the nanny/child lives at this place, we can distinguish among four categories, which are illustrated in Table 3.2. Table 3.3 presents the numbers of each category in my sample.[4]

Live-in nanny is the less common model of delegated childcare in Vietnamese families, as the interviews suggest. In my sample there was only one *live-in nanny* for a limited period. Ms. Lelková started living with a Vietnamese family when they moved to a new house and the distance from the house to her apartment made continuing her caring impossible. The *live-out nanny* is a more common pattern in my sample. Live-out nannies work in the household of Vietnamese families and live in their own households with their husbands and/or children. From all the nannies in my sample, these women had the clearest distinction between private and public, between their own family life and work life. However, as in the case of the *live-out child* (the most common pattern when the care-giving is performed at nanny's place), the distinction is constantly under threat and subject to negotiations between parents and nanny. For instance, nannies complain about the unreliability and unpunctuality of parents who very often come to pick up children later than was agreed. The end of "working hours" is unclear, which not only penetrates into the nannies' lives, but as the nannies stress, is also bad for the children who lack a regular daily routine. *Live-in children* live with their nannies at least five days a week. Some go to their parents' place for the weekend, while some are visited by parents every day of the week/one day in the week at the nanny's place. However, their main residence for a particular period of life is the nanny's home. This model creates the biggest challenge to the nannies' perception of what is home and what is work. At the same time, on the children's part, this model leads to reconsideration of what mothering is (Chapter 4) and how kinship ties are created (Chapter 5).

Besides having time flexibility, these nannies agree to dedicate their time to a job with very low financial compensation. This is possible only for women who have another, official income: i.e. a wage or social wage. In the case of social wages, women in my study received between 6,000 CZK to 10,000 CZK a month.[5] Some nannies (9 out of 15) lived with their partners, and thus were not financially dependent on only their social wage. Nevertheless, being dependent on the welfare state meant a decline in financial status. The official amount of extra money a person dependent on welfare state can earn is limited. A person receiving unemployment compensation may not officially earn any money, while a person receiving a pension or who is on paid maternity or parental leave may earn only

4 My sampling did not reflect the different models so that the differences in the frequency of each model were not purposive.

5 According to Czech Social Security Administration in 2012, the average pension for women was 9,750 CZK (average pension was 10,740; pension for men 11,908), the average pension for woman disability pensioners was 5,699 CZK (average pension was 6,066; pension for men 6,380).

up to a 4,000 CZK a month. Hence, women who want to increase their monthly income must work in the informal labour market, where they have only limited power to negotiate wages. The whole institution of paid childcare here operates in the "off-the-books" labour market, and thus lacks written contracts or any other labour protections.

Keeping in mind that all my nanny-interviewees were dependent on the welfare state, and hence receive limited amounts of money monthly, I assumed that when asking about their motivations to become nannies, I would be told the stories about the family's financial shortcomings. I expected to hear that although the wage for care-giving is quite low comparing to an average salary, it is still a significant financial contribution to the family budget. This was not the case, however. Not all nannies began their stories talking about economic necessity. If they discussed money, it was only to talk about the small things they buy the children, such as candies, ice-cream or Christmas/birthday gifts.

When asked the simple question, "how did you come to be a nanny?," different recruitment logics emerged, most notably in the pattern of who was contacted by whom. Three main models can be observed, which indicate both the strength and weakness of economic motivations in particular cases when (1) the *nanny* finds the job, (2) the *woman* finds the job of *nanny*, and (3) the *family* finds a *woman* and makes her a *nanny.*

Firstly, very few women in my sample were actually trying to find a job as nannies. Ms. Ngoc, mother of two children, told me that a woman had come up to her, asking if she needed a nanny for her child. Even though she was not looking for a nanny at the time, she welcomed the woman who now takes care of their two children. Ms. Ngoc says she was "very lucky" that the nanny had "found" her. Besides directly contacting the Vietnamese family, some women used advertisements to find their employer families. Browsing web pages of advertisements for childcare, I found the ad from Ms. Spáčilová. She wrote that she was on maternity leave and was offering to "take care of children, including Vietnamese ones." I called her to ask whether she had already found a family. Ms. Spáčilová explained why she had decided to place an advertisement, saying that "The mothers who are on maternity leave do it very often; it is normal that they take other children when they stay home with theirs. I wanted to try it too." Another job search strategy was mobilizing social networks. Ms. Jestřábová, who has worked as a nanny for three Vietnamese families, was contacted by two friends of hers, Ms. Kolibříková and Ms. Zvonková. The latter found herself in a bad financial and family situation when her husband became ill, and she had to take care of him. The time requirements for caring for her husband did not allow her to find a job elsewhere, and since she knew about Ms. Jestřábová's job, she decided to ask her for help. Ms. Jestřábová then asked her employers whether some of their friends needed a nanny. A few days later, Ms. Zvonková found her job. Or put more precisely, she found a child to be cared for.

In the second case, when some of my women became dependent on the welfare state, they were forced to look for a job in order to pay the bills. This was the case with Ms. Brhlíková—a disability pensioner in her fifties, mother of three adult daughters,—who suddenly found herself alone as the sole breadwinner. Initially she wanted a job as a shop assistant in Ms. Pham's shop, but when she asked about the job, Ms. Pham replied that she did not need anybody in the shop but did need someone to take care of her baby. "I told her 'she is too small.' She was peeping out from to pram and staring at me. Well, we made an agreement, and that was it," she said. For Ms. Brhlíková, the salary she received for looking after 3-year-old Than (6,000 CZK) doubled her monthly income. For her, caring was an important breadwinning activity. Ms. Křepelková was also looking for a job where she could earn some extra money besides her unemployment benefits. When she saw in a "Vietnamese shop" an advertisement saying "we are looking for someone to watch," she assumed the owners needed somebody to guard the clothes in the shop. When she inquired, they offered her a job looking after a child. In this case, the primary aim was to find a *job*, and this aim was accomplished by finding a job as a *nanny*.

Third, besides the cases of job seekers or nanny-job seekers, there are significant cases of women who were contacted "out of the blue" by families or friends with an offer to become nannies. Contrary to previous women, these nannies-to-be had not been looking for a job. Therefore it was not the demand for job but the external demand for a nanny which led to their decision to accept the job. In these cases, the families find women and make them into workers and nannies. This does not mean these women would not think about taking the job for economic reasons. For instance Ms. Zezulková, a retired teacher at primary school, recalls that when the job was offered to her she did not want to take it because she wanted to enjoy her leisure time, and because she was afraid the children would be a big burden. However, later on she realized that in order to enjoy the leisure, she needed more money than the welfare state gave her each month. She noted that "I knew that I could spend money for a holiday from the wage [for care-giving] which I would not be able to do from my pension." Thanks to her relatively good pension, the decision to become a nanny was determined not so much by the necessity of getting more income, but rather by the protection it afforded her against a lower standard of living after retirement.

To summarize, the importance of economic incentives for becoming a nanny varies among women in my sample. In some cases being a nanny is an indispensable contribution to the family budget, while in others being a nanny provides a little extra money to avoid downward mobility. In addition, a surface reading of their accounts suggests a marginal role for economic motives, which are *retrospectively* denied as the emotional ties between nannies and children develop. Even the nannies whose living standard would be radically lower without the nanny job speak of the secondary role of money in the *paid* childcare they carry out. Ms. Zezulková expresses this in the following words: "So … but the boys grew on me so much that now I cannot imagine not having them. I do not see them one week and I miss them very much because they are just great." Such accounts lead us to consider different sorts of motives which are able to answer the question of why some women that are dependent on the welfare state become nannies in Vietnamese families. What is in it for them? I offer an answer to this question, which I have found when looking at the nannies' caring biographies.

3.2 Creating Caring Biographies: What a Nanny Needs

Being one of the main arenas of doing gender, care work generally and motherhood particularly are considered "a cultural motif that functions to symbolically structure female adult biography" (McMahon, 1995, p.25). Women build their "normal biographies" (Šmausová, 2002) responding to the normative gender orders in which femininity and caring are inevitably entwined. The dialectical relationship between care and femininity lies in the concept that care is gendered as a female activity, and femininity is reaffirmed by the care. Care work, consequently, is considered an activity that requires no qualification but femininity—an extension of what women naturally do (as mothers, sisters, daughters). Accordingly, care work reaffirms the naturalness of the connection between care and femininity.

Prue Chamberlayne and Annette King (2000, p.129) suggest understanding care as a "biographical project, in which past life events and experiences, expectations and aspirations for the future, as well as the present circumstances, are formatively involved in the development of informal care." The authors accentuate that both caring and being a care-giver is actively (re)negotiated and that "caring is an active and potentially transformative process, in which carers need to adjust their perspectives of their own lives to accommodate caring into their own life perspectives" (*ibid.*, p.130). This section builds on Chamberlayne's and King's insight and examines the caring biographies of nannies in order to answer the question of "why do these women work as nannies." Five categories are discussed below, analytically distinguishing different caring biographies according to (1) the past life events and present circumstances that shape the nature of caring biographies at the moment when the woman becomes a nanny for a Vietnamese family, (2) the meaning of paid childcare in the biographies of nannies with regard to their experience, expectations, and aspirations for the future, and (3) general meanings and perceptions of care in the lives of nannies. These categories are not mutually exclusive, and inevitably overlap; however, these distinctions illuminate the importance of the decision to become a nanny in particular (gendered) lives.

3.2.1 Intensification of the caring biography: "I took care of my kids so I simply take other children to look after them"

Ms. Špačková was in her late-twenties when she started taking care of two Vietnamese boys. At that time she lived with her husband and one daughter in one of the housing blocks in Brno, built in the 1970s. Her neighbour—living in the same block of flats—was Ms. Veselá, who soon became Ms. Špačková's friend, and later, her employer (when Ms. Špačková began taking care of Ms. Veselá's sons). The friendship between Ms. Špačková and Ms. Veselá started before both women gave birth to their children. However, the friendship strengthened when they were simultaneously on parental leave. When Ms. Veselá wanted to start working again after her parental leave, she asked her friend and neighbour whether she would take care of her children. This was Ms. Špacková's first experience with paid childcare, which in time would develop into a rich "career" as a nanny to Vietnamese families.

Thanks to Ms. Vesela's relatively prominent position in the Vietnamese community,[6] Ms. Špačková became a much sought-after nanny, and she subsequently worked for five Vietnamese families. She always made her decisions to work as a nanny with regard to her own mothering responsibilities and her children. Following the logic of "I wanted to stay with my children but we needed money," the reasons for becoming a nanny are related to traditional motherhood (Armenia, 2009). I suggest that for Ms. Špačková, paid childcare is understood as a *job* that does not challenge a woman's role as a mother. On the contrary, paid childcare work enables Ms. Špacková to intensify her role as a mother. At the same time, the close interconnection between being a mother and being a nanny means that all recruitment decisions inevitably reflect the needs of the nanny's own children. As she put it, "I took children whose age was similar to my kids so that they all understood each other." Both of Ms. Špacková's daughters (12 and 14 years old at time we met in 2010) grew up with Vietnamese children. When I asked Ms. Špačková if they had ever been jealous, she resolutely denied any such thing, and emphasized that her daughters were so used to this model that the problem (paradoxically), emerged when there was *no* Vietnamese child in their household. She explained how much her two daughters liked all the children she had taken care of, and that once when she had stopped taking care of a little boy, her 2-year-old daughter cried and cried, as he was no longer there to play games with her.

Clearly, as the case of Ms. Špačková indicates, becoming a nanny meant the intensification of a caring biography. This intensification mirrors the logic "I was already looking after my children, so I decided to take on other children." This suggests that for nannies paid childcare is not a job but a natural activity that can be done—with or without salary—while mothering one's own children. Regarding the logic of paid childcare, the cases of women on parental leave are specific in two regards: First, because paid childcare is dependent on and entwined with childcare strategies for one's own children (parental leave), the main aspect defining relationships between nannies and children and their parents is its clear temporary quality. The end of caring is inevitably set by the date when a nanny's parental leave ends and she returns to the formal labour market. Bonds are not developed, and/or they are not supported when care-giving ends. And second,

6 As I have already mentioned above, she was an interpreter, very often contacted by Vietnamese immigrants who need help communicating with the bureaucracy, medical institutions, or even nannies.

for these women the primary goal and driving force for becoming nannies is diversification of income.

3.2.2 Continuation of the caring biography: "I like (taking care of) children"

When I first met Ms. Křepelková in 2010, she was a nanny in her fifth Vietnamese family. Putting together the number of children cared for and the length of time being a nanny, Ms. Křepelková was definitely the most experienced nanny in my sample. I must also add that she was proud of being a care-giver, and during the interview she presented herself as *a very good* care-giver. When talking about the beginning of her nanny-career, Ms. Křepelková explained the roots of her skills as follows:

> I have always had very warm relationship towards children and I have always liked them. I am not trained in childcare or as a teacher, but I have plenty of experience. Since my childhood, it was like a kindergarten in our household (…) I was looking after my siblings, then some children of my relatives and friends. I just liked it.

This account reflects the double-gendered logic of childcare work. On the one hand, Ms. Křepelková's statement demonstrates the role of childcare in her life. In this regard, childcare becomes the main structuring activity of her biography—from childhood when she looked after her siblings, to her work history as a nanny. Her rich care-giving biography was further enriched when her first nanny job launched a chain of subsequent care-giving jobs. Ms. Křepelková was contacted by a number of Vietnamese families who asked her whether she would become a nanny for their children. Many times she had to turn them down; nevertheless, these offers ensured her a steady flow of care work. On the other hand, she considers the work of a nanny as an activity that springs naturally from womanhood and that "is seen as something that women naturally do; it is an extension of their culturally-sanctioned care-giving roles as mothers" (Murray, 1998, p.150).

Ms. Křepelková was not the only nanny in my sample with such extensive experience in paid childcare. Ms. Jestřábová also started her career as a care-giver soon after her parental leave ended. When her parental leave was finished, she found herself unemployed. Then, 10 years later, some Vietnamese parents living in the same area contacted her and asked her to become a nanny. Ms. Jestřábová had not been active in the regular labour market since giving birth to her two children. Ms. Křepelková has also been working as a nanny for more than 12 years. Such long work biographies had an essential impact on their caring biographies, and vice versa. Their extensive experience with (paid) childcare leads to a blurring of work and care-giving biographies. For these nannies, paid childcare is work *with a special meaning*. These meanings are created on the basis of their assumed expertise (which is acquired through practice), and because paid childcare was the main element of their work biographies while they were of productive age.

3.2.3 Diversification of the caring biography: "I cared for my ill husband and I needed to focus my attention elsewhere"

There were three women in my sample who were caring for a dependent family member at the time they decided to become a nanny. Ms. Lelková was already a pensioner when her husband had a stroke and became dependent on her. Ms. Zvonková was in her early forties when her husband developed cancer. Ms. Havranová was a pensioner when her son suddenly became ill and she became a full time care-giver. Taking care of their loved ones was a full-time, round the clock activity for these women, one of whom had to leave the labour market. All three women found themselves isolated in their own households in the role of care-givers. Even if they were receiving financial support for taking care of their ill family members, these women suffered financial difficulties. Meanwhile their opportunities for financial improvement were limited to the four walls of their households. The need for a job in the context of spatial and temporal limitations was perfectly met when the opportunity arose to become a nanny in a Vietnamese family.

However, paid childcare played another, more important role, than that of a mere source of income. Ms. Lelková told me during the interview that her husband had encouraged her to accept the job of nanny. He wanted her to take her mind off things and to focus her attention elsewhere. She remembers how her husband cheered up thanks to the presence of the little boy, who spoke with him and brought new energy into their family. Ms. Havranová reported a similar experience when the health condition of her son was bad and her husband needed to find psychological help. One day, her husband told her: "you know, when the little boy [Chien] put his arms around me and hugs me, it is better than a thousand pills."

It is obvious that paid childcare plays a twofold role in a women's life. As Ms. Zvonková concluded: "I needed money and I was happy that I had these children." For women in this group, taking care of Vietnamese children plays an important psychological role in the nannies' current caring biography, as it helps them deal with the emotional burden of taking care of a seriously ill husband. The nannies see paid childcare as a release, almost a hobby, which makes emotionally exhausting care for a husband more bearable. *Care* for a Vietnamese child becomes a *cure* for Czech nannies. The women then become embedded in the care-giving relationship, which is on the one hand a burden and on the other hand a release.

3.2.4 Compensation of the caring biography: "I was bored and I wanted to experience what I could not experience with my (grand)children"

Early 1998 was a turning point in Ms. Orlová's life: On January 1 she became a pensioner. About two weeks later she brought home a 1-year-old Vietnamese girl named Diu. Ms. Orlová had been living her entire her life in a small village not far from the big Czech city where she worked. Immediately following her studies she had begun working as an accountant in a big factory. When her two sons were born, she stayed home "for a while" on parental leave. After parental leave ended she worked until her retirement. Ms. Orlová's employment history, like those of some other nannies in my sample, was characterized by a lack of time spent with her own children, and later on, with her grandchildren. As she related during her interview: "I could not spend time with them because I had to work. I left in the morning and came back from work late afternoon, so I could not take care of them. So my grandchildren went to kindergarten, and because of my job, I could not help." Here taking care of a Vietnamese child is not just a way to pass the time after retirement, but rather a chance to experience what the nanny could not experience with her own grandchildren, either because she was working, or because the grandchildren lived far away. This reflects the basic logic of the relationship defined above, i.e. that the nanny in the Vietnamese family supplements the mother and supplants the grandmother. In many cases the nanny becomes the primary care-giver for a Vietnamese child, while for her own grandchildren, the nanny is "only" a grandmother (as will be discussed in Chapter 5).

These examples demonstrate another important role of paid childcare in a women's life course. Taking care of a Vietnamese child is experienced as a *rite of passage* from a productive career to retirement. Williams and Baláž (2004) or Búriková and Miller (2010) describe becoming an au pair as the transition between two established stages, as a "lesson in growing up and self-development, a period between living with parents and establishing the conditions for becoming parents" (Búriková and Miller, 2010, p.157). I suggest that the decision to become a nanny is made in order to make the passage from the stage of "being a worker" to the stage of "being a retiree" more bearable. Moreover, for the nannies in this group, taking care of a Vietnamese child has *meant* keeping active; in that sense it is the path to active aging. Taking care of Vietnamese children slows down the process of becoming unproductive, and offers extra time for accommodation to a new life situation.

3.2.5 Completion of the incomplete caring biography: "I miss somebody who needs me. I need to be needed"

Finally, taking care of Vietnamese children as a *rite de passage* from working life to retirement was also significant for the women in this group. If women like Ms. Orlová started taking care of Vietnamese children because of a *lack* of care-giving experience with their own children and grandchildren, for women like Ms. Brhlíková, it was the *absence* of any type of care-giving history that pushed them to become nannies. The *passage* from work life to retirement was accompanied by an inter-generational rupture which left the women alone and/or lonely. For these women, the absence of grandchildren was a crucial formative aspect in their decision to become nannies. However the absence of care-giving differed among women. In the case of Ms. Havranová, this absence was permanent, as she remained childless after her son passed away. In Ms. Brhlíková's case, the absence was temporary, as her own daughters had not had children yet, while Ms. Dudková's relationships with her grandchildren were interrupted.

Inter-generational rupture acquired a different quality in the case of Ms. Brhlíková. When she started caring for Than, she was experiencing the transition between being a "full-time mother" and not yet being a grandmother. Ms. Brhlíková had spent 12 years on maternity and parental leave with her three daughters; hence, taking care of children has been one of her main activities as well as a formative force in her biography. Among the nannies I interviewed, she had the most intensive mothering experience, which not only influenced the way she looked at paid childcare and mothering, but also her decision to become a nanny. A few years ago all her daughters had moved out to live with their partners, and Ms. Brhlíková welcomed this fact as a promise of future growth of her family; she could not wait to become a grandmother. She was therefore very disappointed when one of her daughters started travelling around the world, the second focused more on her career, and the third found a partner who was not interested in having children immediately. During the interviews Ms. Brhlíková complained several times that she longed to be a grandmother, and was sad that her daughters were slow to have children. Evidently her complaints were often verbalized to her daughters. When I spoke with the one daughter who helps her take care of Than, the daughter explained:

> Now she is happy because she has another person she can take care of and who is dependent on her. She is happy for this relationship. We all grew up, we moved away and she used to feel alone and needed to cuddle up to somebody. And she found it here. So it is a kind of compensation for her.

Even though Ms. Brhlíková's daughter used the word "compensation" (she used the same term which I used for previous group of women), I would argue that paid childcare plays a deeper role in her (caring) biography. Depicting their daily routine, she talked about a number of small things she liked about having the responsibility for a little girl. For instance, every day when Ms. Brhlíková comes to the apartment where Than and her parents live, the little girl greets her and waits for the candies her nanny gives every day. The nanny says: "She comes and calls 'granny, granny.' And I cannot help myself, I would give her anything. Well, and I have this complex that I do not have my own grandchildren so that I have to come here to snuggle. She is our baby." The discontinuity in the caring biography, which is experienced when passing from intensive mothering to a (hoped-for) intensive grandmothering, is interpreted by the nanny as her own personal failure. Moreover, it is not only a failing in her care biography, but in her gendered subjectivity. The explicit link between the loss of the intensive mothering experience, and the need to be needed which is fulfilled in the institution of paid childcare, suggests that for Ms. Brhlíková, taking care of Than is inseparable from her negotiation of gendered subjectivity, and is "self-consciously linked to her sense of self and identity" (Chamberlayne and King, 2000, p.131). In other words, to take care of a child is to be a complete person. Ms. Brhlíková defines herself through taking care of children (in the past of her daughters, at present of the Vietnamese girl, and in the future of her grandchildren).

Likewise, Ms. Dudková reported that when she was asked by Ms. Ho to become a nanny for Thuy, she was in a difficult period in her life. Becoming a pensioner was "a big personal crisis in those days," and she missed the active life she had lived as a primary school teacher. The first time she saw Thuy, she said to herself, "we need each other." When Ms. Dudková talked about Thuy it is with love and pride in her voice—both when she enumerated all the skills that little Thuy has thanks to her, and when she talked about how clever and beautiful she is. "I am dependent on her" she told me, and kept expressing the worry that one day Thuy would stop needing her, which would be very painful. Ms. Dudková said that the girl is "a source of energy for her," that taking care of the girl brings her happiness. As in case of Ms. Brhlíková, the emotional interdependence between nanny and child is articulated here.

The emotional investment is reciprocated by the child. For some nannies who cannot have regular face-to-face contact with their grandchildren, their ties with Vietnamese cared-for children serve as a substitute for their emotional loss. In other words, it is not the money they get from care work that is important, but the emotional fulfilment. In case of Ms. Dudková, Ms. Ho and little Thuy, care-giving establishes an emotional win-win score for all three people. Ms. Dudková is able to experience full-time care-giving, which becomes an important structuring factor of her biography; Ms. Ho can rely on Ms. Dudková without worry or stress, and thus focus on providing financially for the family (see Nelson, 1990); and finally, Thuy—who is spoiled by both by her mother and nanny—is well cared for. The emotional win-win is made possible also because the relationship is three-generational: between the "grandmother," Dudková, the mother, Ho, and the daughter, Thuy. Thus the sharing of emotions between Ms. Dudková and Thuy does not challenge Ms. Ho's role as a mother. That is why—in contrast to the findings of many scholars (such as Macdonald, 2010; Lan, 2006)—these nannies do not have to be replaced, and they are not encouraged to employ the rule of detached attachment to protect the mother's exclusive place in the child's life.

During the interviews, these nannies constantly articulated the basic logic of their decision to become a nanny: "to get something that they miss and need." For them, care-giving is a need and makes nannies' lives better. Here, "better" here means complete and valuable. In the words of Wendy Hollway (2006, p.11), "care is the psychological equivalent to our need to breathe unpolluted air. We can survive, perhaps for a long time, in polluted air but it damages our vitality, we have to make do and adapt to less." Care-giving is hence essential for the nanny's female identity work and profoundly structures many women's adult biography (Nelson, 1995). The need to be needed—as evident in the quotation above—indicates that care-giving impacts nannies' self-perception and self-evaluation. To sum up, if for women in the previous category caring for Vietnamese children generated emotions, for women in this category the main outcomes were emotions and, more importantly, self-actualization of gendered biographies and self-definition as women. In addition, while for the nannies in the previous group, paid childcare meant becoming a granny for cared-for children, for nannies in this category it meant becoming a woman again.

In summary, women make their decisions to become nannies on the basis of their caring biographies, and their decisions lead to further enrichment of these biographies. Analysis of their motivations illuminates not only the main incentives leading to the decision to become a nanny, but above all, sheds light on the meanings of (paid) childcare in their lives. I argue that looking at the motivations through this lens enables us to see paid childcare as not just some poorly paid job, but as an activity which plays an important role in their gendered lives. Table 3.4 summarizes the models of caring biographies according to following aspects:

1. the motivations to become the nanny discussed in detail above;
2. the outcomes of paid childcare relationship; i.e. what is the most important achievement for nannies in their paid care-giving history in relation to the motivations;
3. the meaning of care in the caring biographies of women; i.e. how the women perceive childcare, and how they think and talk about paid childcare with regards to their past experiences, expectations, and aspiration for the future.

Table 3.4 Role of paid childcare in nannies' biographies

	Intensification	Continuation	Diversification	Compensation	Completion
Paid childcare motivated by	lack of money	lack of money, love for children	need for activity, lack of money	lack of care-giving	absence of care-giving
paid childcare generates	money and temporary relationships	money and temporary relationships	relationship, emotions and money	long-lasting relationships and emotions	emotions and self-definition
(paid) childcare means	work	work with special meaning	cure and entertainment	being a grandma	being a woman (by being a grandma)

The table illuminates the very distinct trajectories of caring biographies, already apparent at the moment women decide to become a nanny. The broad diversity in motivations, perceptions, and understanding of childcare within the sample of nannies is evident here. The woman's understanding of care shapes the nature of the mother-child-nanny relationship—the employer-employee relationship, but also the kinship ties between nannies and children. Upon examining the nannies' decisions to become nannies in terms of nannies' caring biographies we see that for these nannies, care-giving a Vietnamese child is not a job but rather the extension of care-giving—an activity women normally and normatively have done, now do, and will do in the future. Despite the fact that nannies are paid by Vietnamese parents for care-giving, none of the nannies perceive this activity as *a job*. The nannies usually deny the importance of the financial side of the care-giving, and emphasize that it is an activity which brings them pleasure and fulfillment. Consequently, it is something that the women in my sample *normally* do in various stages of life cycles—as mothers, grandmothers, or care-givers of other family members. As the accounts show, most women at a particular stage of their lives define themselves through the dependence and needs of another person (typically a child but also a grandchild or husband). At the same time it is an activity which they *normatively* do—i.e., they feel they are expected to do according to the normative expectations assigned to female subjectivities (in Czech society).

3.3 Vietnamese Children: Coincidence that Comes in the Right Moment?

In section 2.3 I asked the question of why Vietnamese families hire *Czech* nannies. In this section I ask the question of why Czech women choose to become nannies in *Vietnamese* families. The ethnic aspects of the motivations of Czech women to become nannies for Vietnamese children are often not articulated and, I would argue, even irrelevant for some nannies. This does not mean, however, that the relationship between nannies and families is not marked by ethnic differences and negotiations. Rather these ethnic considerations only come to the fore *after* the decision to be a nanny is made, the woman is already working as a nanny, and when the nanny employs othering strategies. The ethnic logic at the moment of making the decision has two components: first—and most obvious—is the reality of demand; and second—and less obvious—is ethnic stereotyping.

Demand for paid childcare in the Czech Republic is evident in the 1–2 percent of Czech families who seek nannies. In section 2.3 I argued that Czech nannies are "at hand" for Vietnamese families. What is also true is that many Vietnamese families actively seek Czech nannies. As has been already discussed, the majority of nannies were contacted by their future employers. They had not been seeking jobs as nannies, and their decision was usually launched by the logic of "why not?" Regarding their care biographies discussed above, these offers met the needs of women for whom full-time care-giving was the perfect job, one they could not experience if they worked in Czech families. In other words, the specific needs of Vietnamese families (usually full-time caring and passing almost all responsibilities onto the nannies who—at least for a limited period of children's lives—become the primary care-givers) fitted perfectly into the life trajectories of particular women. In addition, taking care of Vietnamese children has become the norm for some Czech women living in a particular area of the Czech Republic with a large Vietnamese population. Several of my interviewees worked as nannies for a number of Vietnamese families in succession. Some of the nannies go from family to family, or are asked whether they have a friend who could take care of friends' children. Experience with taking care of Vietnamese children in some cases sets off a chain of other nanny jobs. Xuan spoke of how much her Czech grandmother cried when she and her brother stopped living with her (they lived with her from Monday to Friday, on weekends with the parents). Soon after they left, the grandma, who lived in western Bohemia (where there is a concentration of young Vietnamese families) began taking care of other small children (much to the anger and jealously of Xuan's brother). According to Xuan the grandma was so accustomed to watching Vietnamese children that she couldn't live without them, as they filled a void she would have otherwise felt.

Hence, as the title of this section suggests, becoming a nanny was for many women a coincidence that came at the right moment, and *from the right person.* This showed up very clearly in the interviews where nannies were asked if they could imagine being a nanny in a Roma or Ukrainian family?"[7] When I asked this question to Ms. Dudková, her partner walked out of the living room, and only came back after she had replied to my question. She explained that her partner did not trust Roma people but that she, as a former teacher, felt children should not be judged by the behavior of their parents. Despite the argument that "all children are nice" (a common remark made by all nannies), my question opened a space for articulating ethnic stereotypes that nannies hold. Ms. Jestřábová referred to Ukrainian immigrants as manual workers, and completely rejected the idea of being a nanny of a Roma child. However, she was not able to explain why, and simply repeated "no, no, I do not know, I simply do not know, I am not racist, but no, no."

The nannies on stereotyping in their decisionmaking, and the positive image these Czech nannies have of Vietnamese, as *distinct* from other minority groups in the country. They emphasized "natural diligence" of Vietnamese parents, which nannies felt was a guarantee that the parents would be hard-working, polite, and caring toward their children, and thus easy to get along with. For many nannies, this would be impossible with Roma parents, who bear the stigma of being unemployed, unadaptable, and generally "problematic." The nannies thus partly base their decisions on the supposition that taking care of Vietnamese children is "unproblematic" because the parents work and their children are high achievers. These images of distinct minority groups reflect the processes of *othering*—ethnicization and classicization—which help nannies differentiate among minority groups, and prefer Vietnamese families. Such rhetoric on the part of the nanny also gives the nanny a sense of autonomy, as she is free to decide whether or not she takes a job.

7 Roma people and Ukranian immigrants are the largest minority groups in the Czech Republic.

When becoming nannies in Vietnamese families, the women start to "love the stranger." In the case of Czech nannies in Vietnamese families, this does not mean just loving *another mother's* child, but a *Vietnamese* mother's child. As I have already mentioned above, the nannies described their ties with children in terms of emotional interdependency. They saw the emergence of emotionality with the child as easy, natural, and spontaneous (see also Macdonald, 2010; Nelson, 1994). "It is impossible not to love them," they stated, referring both to the exceptionality of children (their personal traits, such as beauty, lovability, or brightness), as well as to the simple fact of intensive contact and thousands of hours spent together. This contrasted with their relations with the mothers, which were marked by emotional distance. This distance may be caused by several factors—competition between two care-givers, demonstration of superiority (being the mother and having monopoly control over the child versus being a better care-giver than the working mother)—or may simply be the result of a lack of communication between the two women. However, it is important to mention the impact of emotional interdependence and distance in nannies' understanding of otherness. On one hand, the emotional ties with children serve nannies as a force to overcome their racial prejudices and stereotypes. The *physical* otherness of children is presented in the interviews as something that can be accommodated, erased, or praised. On the other hand, when it comes to mothers, otherness is understood by nannies in *ethnic* terms and usually creates insurmountable barriers between nannies and mothers, which are further nourished by the practices of boundary making—above all with regard to case of mothering strategies (see Chapter 4).

Ms. Brhlíková exemplifies the type of nanny that attempted to *accommodate* to the physical otherness of the cared-for child. Before she started taking care of Than in 2009, Ms. Brhliková received an offer to care for a Vietnamese boy. The offer was tempting, as she was recently retired, and seriously thinking about earning extra money. As she could not make up her mind as to whether to accept the offer or not, she asked a friend for her opinion. The friend told her: "It will be ok now, when he is small. You can put the pram close to the window and open it so that you cannot go outside with him. But what are you going to do when he is three years old or so? Will you put an eye mask on his face [so people do not realize he is Asian] or what?" Ms. Brhlíková seriously considered the offer from the Vietnamese family, but in the end she refused. Nowadays she takes care of 3-year-old Than, and has developed strong bonds with her. To my question "How was the beginning with the little girl?" she answered:

> Nothing, it was normal. She is so cute. But it is true, I don't know whether I should say it, the eyes, I probably should not say it, but I could not get used to it. Well she was sleeping in her pram so step by step I adapted to it. And now I do not care.

As this excerpt demonstrates, the nanny slowly stopped minding the physical difference. It is the establishment of emotional ties between nanny and child which overcomes (but does not erase) what had been a very important aspect—the physical appearance of child. This issue appeared many times during the talk with Ms. Brhlíková, and each time it was rhetorically beaten back by tender words expressing that "yet" she had strong feelings for Than and that she is her "sweet girl."

The second strategy—the *erasure* of the perception of the physical otherness of children—was presented in the interviews when, to my direct question of how it is to be a nanny of a *Vietnamese* child, nannies answered that it is "normal," "they have never had problem with anything" or "children are all the same." The linguistic strategy of erasure may be interpreted as a sign of the nanny's blindness to, or denial of otherness. Such blindness or denial is most likely motivated by the fact that nannies love the children they care for, and know that this question is very sensitive and difficult to talk about. The nannies often deal with verbal or non-verbal attacks on the children—for example when they see that ethnic Czech children do not want to play with the Vietnamese children. These nannies also receive criticism regarding their work as care-givers when they are asked why they do paid care-giving work, and why do it for the Vietnamese. In such a context, denial of any physical otherness or its irrelevance serves to establish the "normality" of their relationship when people point out its "exoticism," and making the "us" and "them" boundaries irrelevant to the nanny-child relationship.

Some nannies in my sample employed the strategy of *praising* the physical appearance of Vietnamese children. Following a line similar to "Black is beautiful," the nannies like Ms. Dudková and Ms. Zezulková kept on saying how beautiful the children are, pointing out the physical traits which according to them distinguish "typical Vietnamese" from "typical Czech." Very often these arguments came together with the nanny's declaration that she "could never be a racist." As such, Ms. Zezulková vehemently rejected the idea that she would ever have a problem with the children's otherness (even during her career as teacher), and offered the following explanation: "I have never had a problem with it. On contrary, these children are so beautiful, they have such wonderful hair. I always say, I would love to have your beautiful black hair because I have curly hair and they have beautifully straight hair. The kids are just scrumptious."

If the strategy of accepting otherness allows nannies to love the children *despite* their physical appearance, the strategy of praising tells nannies to love the children *because of* the difference. Many accounts illuminate how nannies tend to accentuate the advantages of the children's physical otherness, especially in terms of beauty. The strategy of praising the physical appearance shows that physical difference matters in the nannies' perception of the cared-for child. For some nannies, acknowledging the beauty of cared-for child's otherness was an important moment in the interviews, as it was the means to show their openness, and present themselves as tolerant, in contrast to the "racists" around them. The fact that they care for a Vietnamese child is for these women confirmation of their tolerance and lack of prejudice.

* * *

Who can afford to be a nanny in Vietnamese family? Why do women become nannies? And why in Vietnamese families? These questions were dealt with in this chapter. The analysis first looked into the position of these women *vis-à-vis* the welfare state. I have argued that the women's dependence on the welfare state made them suitable candidates as nannies for two reasons: these women have sufficient free time, and lower financial needs, given they receive governmental support, either in the form of unemployment or retirement benefits. For these women, working as a nanny is a job on the side, not the main source of income. Considering the structural position of nannies, I interpreted their decision to become a nanny in the context of their caring biographies, and explored why the nannies *need* paid childcare, and what the value and outcome of (paid) childcare is in their biographies. Only such an analysis can explain the reasoning behind the seemingly irrational decision to work as a full-time nanny for payment far below the minimum wage. As became clear in this chapter, there is an ethnic logic in nanny recruitment—both on the part of families and nannies. However, this logic is very unclear, and very often decisions are not explicitly framed in terms of ethnicity. Ethnicity-based decisions are often muted and become irrelevant, once the relationships have begun to develop. The nannies are unlikely to acknowledge the "otherness" of a cared-for child when deep emotional ties are created. The ethnic framework is only one piece of the puzzle, and has only supplemental explanatory value. The Vietnamese families seek *nannies*, and they hire *Czech* nannies because they are available and willing to work for them. Czech women tend not to be looking for nanny jobs, but are contacted by families that offer them work as nannies. These families happen to be Vietnamese. So in response to the questions why Vietnamese families recruit *Czech* nannies, and Czech women work in *Vietnamese* families, the answer could be put as: Why not?

3.4 Provisional Conclusions to Chapter 2 and Chapter 3: Mutual Dependency and the Puzzles of Motivations

Julia Wrigley (1999, p.169) writes in her article on hiring the nannies in the USA that "care-givers and parents have minimal formal obligations to each other, but care-giving arrangements can entail high levels of dependency." As we have seen so far, mutual dependency on the micro level (that is, what families need and how their needs are met in nannies' biographies and *vice versa)*, exists in a specific structural context that provides both nannies and families with a basic set of options and patterns for childcare arrangements. From the structural point of view, the relationship of delegated childcare is conditioned by the interplay of exclusions and inclusion from/in the labour market, where inclusion and exclusion operate in mutual relation to each other and enable the emergence of the relationship.

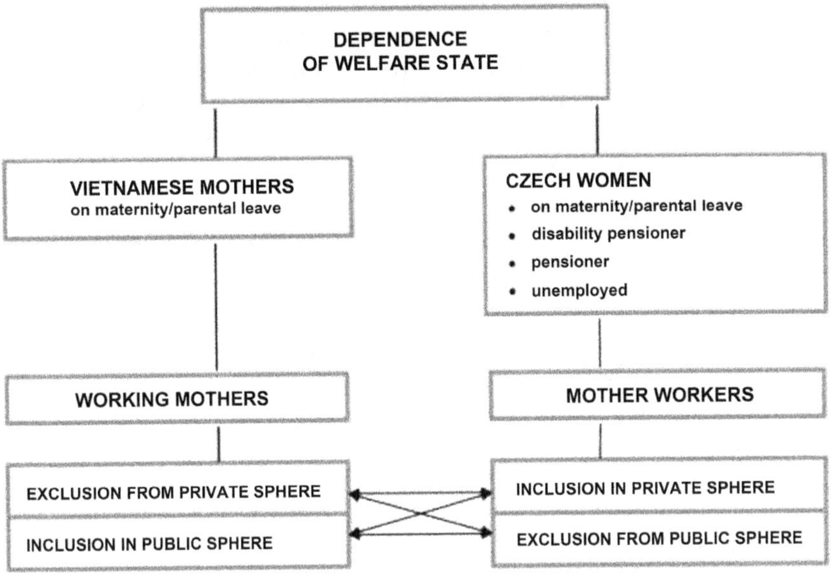

Figure 3.1 Mutual relations of exclusions and inclusions

The diagram illustrates the basic mutuality of relations between Vietnamese (working) mothers and nannies (mother workers) on the boundary between public and private. It shows that inclusion in the public sphere (incorporation on the labour market) of one woman and her (self-)exclusion from the private sphere is possible only when another woman is simultaneously excluded from the public sphere (from the workforce) and included in the private sphere (as a nanny performing her job in her or her employer's household). It is the Vietnamese mother who returns to work, along with her husband or under her husband, while her child is cared for at home by a nanny who cannot or does not want to be included in the public sphere and hence the regular labour market. The nanny's inclusion in the private sphere where she is paid to work as a care-giver, means the illegalization of the whole relationship when the nanny works "inside the family, and outside of labor law" (Macdonald, 2010, p.45).

This illegalization allows women on both sides to actively work and do their best to profit the most. Illegalization is not interpreted as a drawback of the care work constellation, but rather as the very condition enabling the relationship to be established. At the same time, the shared consciousness of illegality of the employer-employee relationship may serve as grounds for mutual trust. Illegalization establishes *an alternative space of resistance to the welfare state*, which is manifested in the contract between the welfare-state-dependent nannies, and mothers who do not want to be dependent on the welfare state. First, on the side of the nannies, it generates demand for extra money (as the social wages are not sufficient) and extra activity (as retirement is understood as a life stage of unproductivity and inactivity). Secondly, on the part of the parents, there is demand for a private solution to childcare, which the state (with its declining support for public childcare institutions) does not provide. It is the failure of the welfare state that provides both parties to the care-giving contract with a perfect space for creating their relationship to one another. These relationships are marked by the disadvantages associated with the irregular labour market—lack of security, regulations, unclear boundaries of work, uncertainty of work hours. However I would argue that, in the end, it is the welfare state which profits most from such childcare arrangements. First, it relieves the state of the responsibility of having to provide public support for childcare, as the responsibility for childcare is transferred from the state to the parents. Second, nannies act as a bridge between the Vietnamese community and mainstream Czech society. Delegated care work thus relieves the state of the additional burden of having to integrate second-generation immigrant children into the educational system and society in general. The burden of integration projects is removed from the state, as this becomes one of the main tasks of the nannies, who prepare children for kindergarten and serve as the "door to majority" for children of immigrant parents (see Chapter 4).

Thinking about the motivations for becoming and hiring a nanny within the mainstream framework is quite difficult, as the dominant scholarship is usually based on case studies of immigrant nannies working in (upper) middle-class families. As we have seen, paid care is not necessarily the privilege of rich Western families alone (as the concept of global care chains suggests). It is also a necessity for families that find themselves in a particular economic and social situation—such as for these Vietnamese families after migrating to the Czech Republic. At the same time, the incentives for Czech women to become nannies in Vietnamese families challenge the assumption that the economic aspect of *paid* childcare is the main driving force. I argued that we must understand their motivations to become part of the paid childcare relationship in the context of their caring biographies. In other words, it is not "paid" childcare that attracts these women, but rather paid child "care." Therefore, I have suggested that we should see these motivations through the lens of mutual dependency, which allows us to contemplate how motivations on one side complement motivations on the other side, and vice versa. Simply put, the motivations to recruit nannies are found in the post-migratory family constellation, where the grandmother—, as the usual support for childcare in Vietnam,—is missing. The motivations to become nannies, on the other hand, can be found in the caring biographies of these nannies, and their intergenerational relationships. This general logic is crucial for understanding the complexity of relations and kinship ties, as well as tensions and ambivalences (as will be discussed in the following chapter).

Chapter 4
"Everything for Us but Nothing with Us": The Meaning of Motherhood, Delegation of Care Work and its Consequences

> All mothers in the world love their children.
>
> Ms. Duong, mother of two children

> I admire them in the sense that they are able to put such little children to a stranger, to a person that they do not know at all. And they go back to work. Well, I would not have heart and stomach for that.
>
> Ms. Zvonková, nanny of two Vietnamese girls

My name is Linh and I am 20 years old. I was born in Vietnam and when I was seven months old, we moved to the Czech Republic. After we came here, my mum had to start working, so I had my first Czech family I lived with. And then we moved to another town; there I was living with my Czech nanny and her husband. They are my Czech grandparents. At the beginning I was only with them during the day, and in the evening my parents picked me up and we went home. But when I was six years old, my parents decided to move to Prague and try their luck there. They knew that it would be very difficult at the beginning for them so they left me at my grandma's. My parents came to see me from time to time, or I went to them like for a holiday, or we spent Christmas together.

I could not spend much time with my parents—that is why my upbringing looks like it does. My grandparents pampered me very much. I had a nice childhood with them, I had everything. Every day I when woke up, my breakfast was already prepared; when I came from school, my lunch was ready and after writing homework I could do whatever I wanted. When I brought a D grade from school, my granny said "It's ok, it's better than an E!" So I did not have a strict Vietnamese upbringing—I had freedom, no pressure on school aspirations, no obligations about housework. So this is how I lived until the age of 10. And then everything changed.

Suddenly, one day my parents decided to take me back to live with them in Prague. It was cruel. I still remember how on the first day at home I was awakened at seven in the morning by my mother who told me: "we go to work, we come back around 10 pm, so you must prepare lunch, iron the laundry, clean, and look after your 2-year-old brother." And that was it. I had no idea how to do these tasks because I was so young. In addition, I considered it unfair that I suddenly became responsible for the household tasks, because my friends did not have to do anything. I felt wronged but step by step I learnt how to do the household chores. I was calling my granny all the time, and for her it was also very hard because she missed me so much. I know that she was begging my parents to let me live with them, not to take me from them, she even said that they did not have to pay for it, she would do it because she loved me.

The biggest problem was that I did not understand my parents at all. I knew only the basic vocabulary and our perception of reality was so different! It took us eight years to find the way back to each other because they did not comprehend my thinking and I did not comprehend theirs. For example, I was used to the open manifestation of love and emotions which my grandparents made; they were hugging me and kissing me all the time and kept on saying how great I was and how much they loved me. I think this is how it works in the Czech families. My parents seemed cold. Well, it was really hard for both of us, there were no emotional ties. I did not regard them as my parents and they did not consider me as their child. We did not know anything about each other. All in all, moving to my parents was a big shock for me. Not only did I have to do everything around the household, but also they pushed me to study more, to be the best in everything. My nanny was not that strict in this—I was used to doing my homework, of course, but then I could play. But with my parents, I had to attend some additional courses. I know that they did it for my own good, but I do not think this is the best way to up bring your child.

Actually, you can imagine my personality as the fusion of two persons—one who was brought up in a Czech family by a Czech granny, and the other raised by Vietnamese parents. The first one's name is Linda (this is how my Czech family called me and I still use this name for my Czech friends). She is not practical at all; she cannot move a finger in the household. Well, maybe to prepare tea, that is all. She is very friendly, carefree, and on the menu she finds the cheapest thing and complains about how everything is expensive. The second one's name is Linh and she is the top pupil. And she cannot sit in the café because she must study hard, have private lessons in English or something. She is less open and more cold. And she definitely does not speak with Linda. So here I am, two in one, one in two!

* * *

The story of Linh is presented here as a point of departure for the analysis of the mothering strategies, delegation of care work and its consequences for mothers, nannies, and children. Linh's story is the most polarized among the accounts I heard from the children in my sample. It is not a typical case within my sample, but rather one that reflects all the issues and consequences of care work delegation, which appear separately in all the interviews.

This chapter focuses on how mothers, nannies, and children reflect upon the care contract and their positions and roles within the delegation of care work. As the story of Linh (as a live-in child) shows, a large number of activities are transferred (i.e. not shared) from parents to nannies. In many cases the outcome of this transfer is that the nanny becomes (for a certain period of child's life) the child's primary care-giver. As the age of cared-for children varies from a few weeks to several years, and because the relationship between nanny and family is very often long-term, the exact activities nannies are supposed to do vary over time. Some nannies are hired as nurturers, while others could be characterized as "teachers," as their main task is to pick up the child from school or kindergarten and spend the time with her/him doing homework or playing games before the parents come home from work. In addition, in cases where the relationship is long-lasting, both roles are combined—the nanny may toilet train a child one year, and a few years later, help the child with his homework. Becoming the primary care-giver, or at least the only care-giver with knowledge of the Czech language, means that another of the nanny's tasks is to negotiate with social institutions, such as health care and education. Accompanying children to the doctor, and being the main contact person for the children's teachers, the nanny extends her care-giving role beyond the home. This role is in turn recognized and accepted by persons outside the household—such as teachers, school directors, doctors, etc. Many—if not all—of the nannies in my sample were involved in the decision-making about the child. As the nanny spends more time with the child than any other adult, and is the principle repository of knowledge regarding Czech culture and society in the Vietnamese household, her opinions about the child's welfare (such as schooling) are highly valued and necessary.

Delegation of childcare establishes the relationship between two women, usually two mothers who enter the relationship with their own ideas, ideals, and experiences of mothering. These ideas and experiences vary according to their particular socio-cultural and historical context. Differences in mothering strategies have been discussed in many studies—particularly those focusing on delegated childcare (Macdonald, 2010), migrant women's motherhood (Erel, 2009; Lutz, 2011) or the motherhood of black/minority women (Collins, 1994; Segura, 1994, and so on). This scholarship has challenged the universal notion of motherhood, and shown that women performing alternative forms of mothering have to struggle with a commonsense understanding of good motherhood, which continues to draw upon the western image of at-home motherhood.

These issues will be dealt with in the following two sections of this chapter, which focuses on Vietnamese mothering strategies and Czech nannies' perceptions of motherhood. In the third section, the delegation of motherhood is analyzed from the point of view of the children, focusing on how they comprehend the delegation of care and how this delegation impacts their understanding of inter-generational ties and the notion of family. It has become quite common in the scholarship on care work to discuss the clash of mothering strategies between nannies and mothers (as Macdonald did in 2010, brilliantly); however, it seems to be forbidden to ask children about their interpretation of care-giving (see Prout and James, 1997). The main starting point for the analysis presented in this section is that children are active agents in their upbringing. They create their own identities, select the influences of socialization, and shape their own perspectives on social phenomena and institutions. Balancing these three perspectives, the chapter illuminates another level of mutual dependencies in the nanny-mother-child ties: mutual dependency in mothering strategies.

4.1 The Labour Market as a Post-Migratory Site for Doing Motherhood

Ms. Ho is a mother of two children. In the 1990s she followed her husband to the Czech Republic where they started their business. Reflecting on her arrival to Europe, she told me: "When I moved here, I had the vision that we would earn money and bring up our kids in a better environment. After all, they have more opportunities here." Ms. Ho sold clothes together with her husband in their shop, and found a nanny when their children were only couple of months old. The family's financial situation did not allow the mother to remain at home with the children. Ms. Ho's contribution to the family business was important for the future of their children, as it brought the economic capital necessary for the children's education and subsequent incorporation into the labour market. Ms. Ho told me: "For us, the most important thing in raising children is to direct them so that they try hard. In everything. We are foreigners here, and it will be difficult for them [the children] to prove that they are not worse than other people. We want them to have a better life than we currently have." To ensure this, Ms. Ho mobilized her efforts in the labour market while her children were with a nanny.

The example of Ms. Ho demonstrates how Vietnamese mothers in my sample understand their role as mothers, which they see as providing sufficient economic capital in order to ensure greater opportunities and a better future for their children. Following this argument, this section will further develop the argument already formulated in Chapter 2. There I argued that Vietnamese parents' migration is defined as oriented towards children and that parents hire Czech nannies in their effort to simulate typical childcare arrangements in Vietnam. In this section I will examine how the delegation of motherhood becomes a way of doing "good motherhood." After looking into how mothers delineate their responsibilities *vis-à-vis* their children, this section reveals their definition of care-giving and mothering in relation to their breadwinning activity.

4.1.1 Good Mothering as Providing "Better Tomorrows"

Ms. Ho, as well as other interviewees, singles out education as a main objective of childrearing, and emphasis on education as one of the key differences between Vietnamese and Czech childrearing practices. Vietnamese interviewees consider Czech childrearing to be more "benevolent," and Vietnamese childrearing more "goal oriented." Many studies show that Asian immigrant parents play a critical role in their children's education, and have high expectations of academic success on the part of their children (Kao, 1995). An inspiring contribution to this debate was made by Pranee Liamputtong (2006, p.42). She focuses on how migrant mothers define themselves as "good mothers," and shows that "Children's education played an important part in being a good mother. A good mother (…) needed to provide good education and support to her children, so that the children's future would be positive." This is echoed in interviews with mothers, such as Ms. Duong, mother of two children: "The most important thing for their future is their studies. When they study, they will have an academic degree so it will be easier for them to find a job anywhere. Especially in Vietnam, if they wanted. So now they must study a lot."

Achieving education and finding a job appear in the interviews as a reply to challenges brought to the children's by the parents' migration. Consequently it is the task of a good mother to mobilize and motivate her children to make use of the conditions pre-prepared by their parents' arrival in the Czech Republic and their economic activity. The children live in Europe so that they can get a "European education" which is valued more than an Asian one. At the same time children are provided by their parents with the economic capital necessary to get a superior education. Good mothers, the Vietnamese mothers told me, must encourage their children's studies (by paying for extra lessons in language school, in mathematics, etc.) and hobbies (such as art lessons). Paying for private education, additional courses after school, or holidays in English-speaking countries—all financially burdensome activities—are considered by mothers to be the main ways to give their children the best education possible.

Mothers believe their children should get the best education possible in order to overcome two kinds of stigma that their children face: first, the stigma of being "foreigners"—the good mothers bring up children who are included in the majority—, and second, the stigma of being a "stallholder"[1]—the good mothers bring up children who find their job outside the immigrant economy. In both cases, education is meant to ensure social mobility, and to overcome the barriers between "them" and "us." In the first case, the borders are defined in ethnic terms, and in the second case in generational terms. The mothers stress educational success, which serves as proof that their children are not worse than others (meaning people from the majority). Improvements in their status and work position can be attained mainly by cultivating cultural capital. Vietnamese mothers experience what Macdonald observed in upper-middle class American families, where some mothers are under the pressure of competitive mothering and the children are directed to elite pre-schools, elementary and high schools, and universities. Macdonald (2010, p.35) writes that in such cases, "being a good mother frequently meant working to fund these enrichment activities, at the same time that working outside of the home often felt like being inadequate as a mother." Such inadequacy is willingly acknowledged in the interviews with nannies (see below).

Achieving education is far from being only an individual matter or just the success of the child. In Vietnamese culture, a child's education reflects a family's

1 Many children encounter the general stereotype in which the Vietnamese is equated with stallholder and stallholder means unqualified.

status, and is thus extremely important (see also Kibria, 1993). The accent on education is very much emphasized in interviews with children. Anh, a 23-year-old university student, in concurrence with others, made an explicit link between the intensification of work life, earning money, and considering children's education as the main achievement of migration. She concluded that "first the status symbol was the money; then money was not enough so it was a modern car, and now because everybody has a car, it is the children." Like Anh, Khanh also talked about the big celebration her parents prepared when she successfully passed her secondary school exit exams. Many friends and distant kin members were invited to celebrate her school success, even though she protested that it was too expensive and pointless. For her parents on the other hand, it was an important event, demonstrating the family's social status, attained through their child.

The success of a child becomes a symbol of a prestige of the whole family in the Vietnamese community. That is why the mothers in the interviews spent a lot of time bragging about their children and their plans for the future. Attaining education by a particular family member becomes a collective family project and once it is attained, it becomes the victory of the whole family. In this view, second generation children are responsible for the wellbeing of three generations: the parents who sacrificed their lives and moved to the Czech Republic, the second generation children themselves who thanks to their parents could build a good position in the Czech Republic, and their children who will be born to already integrated offspring of first generation immigrants.

4.1.2 Against the Dichotomy of Care Versus Work: Care-Giving as Breadwinning

To follow this definition of motherhood in a new country, the mothers must invest a lot of energy and time into breadwinning activity. However, this is not a new phenomenon caused only by migration. Rather, breadwinning activity is part of how normal caring biographies are understood in Vietnam. And this understanding entails three crucial aspects: First—regarding the frequency of informal childcare delegation (usually to grandparents)—we see that non-singular mothering practices are normative in Vietnam where Vietnamese mothers were mothered. Second, mothering is not based on physical proximity, even when the children are only a few months old. And third, as family policy is meant to encourage the quick return of mothers to the work force, the role of mother as a breadwinner is common, and is a mark of a normal caring biography. However, as became evident in the previous section, the post-migratory situation of families makes the accent on working even stronger. Ms. Ngoc, a mother of two children, balanced the difference between mothering and working in Vietnam and in the Czech Republic by saying: "Life is hard here. If just one of us worked, we would not have enough money for bread and butter. That is why we had to find a nanny, because we both needed to work."

Vietnamese parents create dual-earner households and harmonize work and childcare by delegating childcare to nannies. The duality of care-giving and breadwinning becomes an everyday issue here, and "harmonizing" means radically different things for Vietnamese mothers, for nannies, and for children. Nannies and some children—as the following text will show—understand care and work as a dichotomy, as "either-or." Consequently these nannies and children are critical of Vietnamese mothers, whom they feel do not fulfil the normative ideal of motherhood, in which integration into the labour market is incompatible with being a good mother. This view is shaped by the experiences of women that are socially *privileged* enough to be able to be "stay-at-home" mothers (Segura, 1994; Arendell, 2000). However, this is not the case for Vietnamese immigrant mothers. As is apparent from the definition of care-giving that Vietnamese mothers "bring" from Vietnam, "at-home" mothering is not a common pattern, and breadwinning activity is not in opposition to care-giving. On the contrary, breadwinning is considered by Vietnamese mothers to be an essential part of care-giving.

Feminist scholars focusing on the practices of motherhood at a distance (Erel, 2009; Lutz, 2010; Chamberlain, 1997), or on migrant and working mothers' mothering (Liamputtong, 2006) have called for acknowledging the breadwinning role of mothers as an integral part of "good mothering," and not as a mark of a woman's failure as a mother. Addressing the barriers that working mothers must overcome to attain high marks in mothering practices, Liamputtong (2006, p.45) writes: "Good mothering needs time and energy to care for children. Due to the physically demanding nature of their [immigrant or poor mothers'] work, it is difficult, or even impossible, to be a 'good mother.'" As Bridget Anderson (2000, p.118), suggests:

> migrant women can have little emotional and moral input into the upbringing of their children. They do not enjoy care as emotion freed from physical labour. Instead the opposite applies: their care for their children is demonstrated in the fruits of hard labour, in remittances, rather than in cuddles and 'quality time' that provide so much of the satisfaction of care.

Such studies contribute to a redefinition and expansion of the notion of 'the good mother' that moves beyond 'the sacrificial mother' to include working as a way of supporting the family economically" (Macdonald, 2010, p.6). Similarly, Vietnamese mothers do not understand the duality of work and care as either a dichotomy or as mutually exclusive. For Vietnamese mothers, work and care are in harmony—the latter is accomplished through the former—and being a mother and a worker does not imply a conflict of roles. The work ethic of Vietnamese mothers is not based on the ideas of self-realization, but on providing children with the economic capital that the children are supposed to then turn into cultural capital. The family is primarily an economic unit meant to support social upward mobility for the next generation, and to ensure prosperous post-migratory lives. That is why it is more important for mothers to work and earn money for the future of their children than to be socially and emotionally present in their children's everyday lives. Motherhood is not in opposition to working in the labour market. On the contrary, the labour market is the arena where motherhood is performed through breadwinning activity. To fulfill their ideal of motherhood, Vietnamese mothers become dependent on Czech nannies, who care for their children at home, while the mothers themselves care for their children through their work in the labour market.

* * *

In Chapter 2, I argued that Vietnamese mothers' motivations for hiring nannies is a response to changes brought on by migration, and that Vietnamese families simulate the model of care common in Vietnam when they hire a nanny. In this section I go a step further by arguing that delegated care-giving is an essential part of "good motherhood" as defined by Vietnamese mothers. This delegation of motherhood enables Vietnamese mothers to be good mothers, which means forming part of the labour market through breadwinning activity. Providing their children with economic capital, the mothers provide their children with a better future in which the children overcome both the stigmas of being a "stallholder" and a foreigner. Having a child that attains the best possible education and a good position in the labour market, proves to the mothers that their "migration project" was successful, and their motherhood practices were well performed.

4.2 Moral Hierarchies as a Defense of the Nannies'/Czech Mothering Strategies

Nannies enter relationships with children and mothers with their own cultural ideas and ideals about mothering. There were two distinct types of women-mothers in my sample regarding their mothering strategies and their ideals about how motherhood should be performed: working mothers who brought up their children before 1989, and full-time mothers who had their children after 1989 in the era of re-familization (Sirovátka and Saxonberg, 2006; see Chapter 4). As Hana Hašková pointed out, while in the 1960s 75 percent of mothers stayed home with their children for up to two years (of which 61 percent stayed a maximum of one year), in the 1990s only 22 percent did so. In addition, 51 percent of women stayed home for between two and three years, and 27 percent stayed home even longer than three years (Hašková, 2005). It is apparent that there exist two distinct periods and ideologies of care in which the nannies brought up their children. These shaped their understanding of what a "normal caring biography" is and how "good motherhood" should be performed.

Eight of the 15 nannies in my sample brought up their children in the pre-1989 era. All eight share a common characteristic of their motherhood—all of them were *working mothers*. Recalling their motherhood experiences, nannies described two elementary characteristics of mothering during the communist era: all women worked, and a well-developed system of childcare existed. Hence, for these nannies, the roles of mother and worker were performed simultaneously and harmoniously thanks to state support, and the general belief that mothering and outside employment are reconcilable and compatible. Experience with working double shift equipped these nannies with partial pre-comprehension of Vietnamese working mothers. Seven of the 15 women in my sample were *full-time mothering mothers*. Compared to the previous group, these interviewees described their mothering ideals and experiences in terms of "enjoying motherhood" and staying with the children as long as possible. Some of them took advantage of the extended periods of parental leave established by post-communist governments in early-1990s, and were able to stay home up to four years with each child. As most of them had more than one child, the total length of their at-home mothering could reach eight years or even more. These nannies bear witness to the process of re-familization, and to the emergence of an intensive mothering ideology that promotes stay at-home mothering and strict polarization of gender roles between breadwinners and care-givers.

However, despite differences in their own mothering experiences, all the nannies were critical of the Vietnamese mothers' mothering strategies. *Leaving* the child with another woman was something they (the nannies) would never do (and never had to do)—either because they could rely on state supported nurseries or because they themselves could stay at home. In both cases, their position as a mother and primary care-giver remained secure. Espousing the ideal of intensive mothering—with its accent on the primacy of one care-giver (the mother)—these nannies (unconsciously) undermined their own position in the relationship with the child, and partly devaluated their role of a care-giver (Macdonald, 2010). They did so when employing moral hierarchies, judgments about a mother's mothering (Uttal, 1993 in Uttal and Tuominen, 1999). These moral hierarchies played an essential role in nannies' relations with and attitudes towards Vietnamese mothers, but also with their self-definitions as mothers, as I will show in the following lines.

To properly understand the role of moral hierarchies, one must first answer the questions as to how nannies understand "moral" and "hierarchical." To do so, I use a statement appearing repeatedly in the interviews with nannies (see also the quotation of Ms. Zezulková at the beginning of this chapter): "How can she leave her little child? I could not do it." The first half of the statement—"How can she leave her child?"—refers to a commonly discussed aspect of (delegated) childcare and mothering: that the institution of paid childcare violates the ideal of motherhood and challenges the mother's womanhood. As McMahon (1995, p.24) succinctly puts it: "motherhood is constructed as the expression of women's natural, social, and moral identity—or, rather, the identity attributable to moral women, that is married white women." Under the ideology of intensive mothering, care and childcare is coded as a naturally female activity enacted in a female-coded realm of the private sphere and, as Helma Lutz argues, is a core activity of doing gender (Lutz, 2008c). Womanhood is entwined with and defined through caring. As became apparent in Chapter 3, where the caring biographies of nannies were discussed, mothering and care-giving are essential parts of a woman's moral identity—and this is what makes moral hierarchies *moral.* Understanding mothering as the expression of female gender identity impacts how nannies view Vietnamese mothers' mothering strategies—usually described in terms of failure, lack or absence. As Margaret K. Nelson (1994, p.182) writes: "if care is the work a woman is compelled to do, it is also an essential component of her identity." In other words, to be a woman, a woman must mother. A mother that delegates childcare fails as a mother and as a woman. Such a mother displays her lack of femininity, and fails "at one of the primary responsibilities of adult womanhood" (Macdonald, 2010, p.25). If failing as a mother means failing as a woman, then conversely, being a good care-giver means being a good woman. Moral hierarchies serve nannies to display this dialectic.

"I could not do it," forms the second half of the argument, often echoed in my interviews when it came to judgments about the way the mothers demonstrate their motherhood. It was their point of departure to make the morality of motherhood strategies hierarchical. The nannies I interviewed explicitly or implicitly defined themselves as better care-givers (mothers and nannies) than their employers. The sources of this self-presentation were the age of the nanny, her experience with mothering, and her experience with mothering in the Czech Republic. All the nannies in my sample (with one exception) were older than the mothers, and this seniority in the employer-employee relationship made them more experienced both as human beings and as care-givers. More experienced nannies consider themselves more capable care-givers, who can provide children with superior care and hence raise them better than the children's parents ever could. The nannies view themselves as more skilled in care-giving, and to prove it they point out that the children behave better with them than with their parents (see also Macdonald, 2010). The nannies' "expertise" in child rearing was further strengthened by their ethnic background (elaborated in more detail later in this section). All in all, this led to the definition of the "ideal" by which all mothering practices are to be measured. This ideal was compatible with the nannies' experiences of mothering in the Czech Republic, while Vietnamese mothers in many respects deviated from such an ideal. During the interviews with nannies, it was clear that the nannies' evaluation of Vietnamese mothers' mothering was also a self-evaluation of the nannies' own mothering and caring strategies. Moral hierarchies provide nannies with the opportunity to define themselves as better care-givers, and many nannies make use of this. Nannies who had mothered after 1989 were particularly critical of working mothers and paid childcare. These nannies, as Margaret K. Nelson states on the basis of her own research, "allow other women to be mothers in a manner they personally find unacceptable" (Nelson, 1994, p.192). Paradoxically, nannies with experience of being working mothers (before 1989) were also critical of the working mothers they worked for. However, they were able to acknowledge the socio-historical and economic context of the decision to return to the labour market.

Having described the logic of moral hierarchies, we must turn now to their manifestations. They differ according to the nannies' attitudes towards mothers, the intensity of direct criticism and the level of the nannies' agency to impact on mothers' mothering. Hence, in the accounts I distinguish three approaches to judging mothers' mothering strategies: the nannies as open critics, as teachers, and as boasting care-givers.

The first, and mostly employed, strategy to articulate moral hierarchies was to become "open critics." The mothers were criticized for a variety of reasons, most commonly for working, and for supposedly being too "ambitious" and "cold." Vietnamese mothering strategies are rated low on the nannies' scale of moral hierarchies, and attributed to the otherness of these mothers as Vietnamese.

The nannies' criticism of *working* mothers was motivated by the assumption that working and mothering are incompatible, and that a good mother will always choose mothering over working (see also Uttal and Tuominen, 1999). The idea that motherhood and employment are irreconcilable—especially in the case of pre-school children—is related to the nannies' own caring biographies, and to the ways they performed their own motherhood. Nannies with the experience of full-time mothering were especially critical of the mother's decision to work. In this regard, the nannies criticisms of the mothers' employment decisions were unanimous about the extent to which the mother's decision was driven by real necessity. The nannies reported that the mothers wished to return to work out of personal desire rather than out of economic necessity. Interpreted as the "*decision* to *leave* the child" (voluntarily give up childrearing), the nannies see the Vietnamese mothers' strategies as exhibiting a lack of interest in childcare and a muted (or even absent) "maternal instinct." Therefore the nannies do not dare to ask, like Ms. Křepelková, "why do they have children at all?" referring to the lack of interest in being proper (meaning at home and full-time) parents. Paradoxically, the tensions generated here have the same source—the idea of self-sacrifice for the children—that motivates both radically different ways of caring, both being subjectively recognized as the mark of good motherhood. For the nannies, the sacrifice for children means giving up career/work life for family life and raising children. For Vietnamese mothers, on the other hand, the core element of this sacrifice is an intensive work life lived *for* the children, but not necessarily *with* the children.

As noted above, the most important aim and indication of a Vietnamese mothers' good mothering skills are the child's educational achievements, as these will lead to child's successful integration into the Czech labour market and society. Observing these efforts of the parents, the nannies were critical towards the parents' stress on education, and criticized the mothers for being *too ambitious*. There were two particular reasons for the nannies' criticism of parents' ambitions. First was the discrepancy between the time the parents spent with their children, and the parents' requirements of them. The nannies pointed out what they considered the inappropriateness of working outside *just* to pay for additional education at the expense of spending time with the children. The second reason was that the nannies felt that the demands on the children were exaggerated, described as "too much" or inappropriate for the children's upbringing. The "wrongness" of Vietnamese parental pressure is seen both in relation to the child's own needs—when the children had to attend additional classes for much older students because their parents wanted them to know more and be better than their schoolmates—, and in contrast to the nannies' own children—who were lower achievers than Vietnamese children. In both cases, the nannies reported that they felt sorry when seeing the Vietnamese children stressed and missing out on a "carefree childhood." The example of this kind of moral hierarchy illuminates a clash of ideals not only regarding motherhood, but regarding childhood, as well. For the mothers, childhood is a period of preparation for successful adulthood, and must be filled with educational achievements. For the nannies, on the other hand, childhood should be a time of games and care-free living.

Lack of time spent with children, and excessive pressure on education went hand in hand with mothers' lack of emotional demonstrativeness toward their children. Many nannies considered themselves providers of emotions—giving the children not only daily care, but also the love the mother does not provide. Referring to the symbiosis of the nanny-child unit, the nannies described their relation to children in terms of mutual emotionality (see Chapter 3), and give many examples of what "cold mothers" do and do not do. They do not hug the child; they are not interested in what the child does beyond school achievements, the nannies say. In this sense, the nannies declare their *emotional superiority* over the mothers. What the nannies interpreted as "cold," the children and mothers perceived as "strict" (with both positive and negative connotations). Mothers saw themselves as strict because for them being strict was the way to motivate children to become good persons—to be educated, decent, respectful and obedient to parents. As Umut Erel (2009, p.126) argues, "other mothers [read here: nannies] may be able to provide for the emotional needs of children, precisely because they do not have the burden of providing economically for them." Many of the children responded in similar fashion. Trai reported that "parents cannot provide for us a family life because they must provide for us financially."

The second strategy employed by nannies is what I call "nannies as teachers." The nannies took upon themselves the (unsolicited) task to assist mothers with improving their mothering strategies and becoming better mothers. By so doing, the nannies create and shoulder the burden of a being a good mother, while at the same time teach "bad" mothers how to mother. The nannies thus make themselves responsible for the mother's mothering and mother's "reorientation" towards good or at least better motherhood. Here we can observe three "lessons" in mothering: when nannies teach mothers the physical contact with children; family activities; and childcare responsibilities.

The *lesson in physical contact* is taught when the nanny does not agree with the lack of time parents spend with children, and she interferes in their organization of daily routine. An unconditional order came from Ms. Kosová, the nanny of a live-in child. Her lesson given to the parents at the very beginning of her care-giving was clear and unprecedented. "I told them: 'you will come here so that you know you have a kid.' If I had told them: 'you don't have to come if you don't care,' maybe they would not have come at all." Anticipating that the parents would not come, Ms. Kosová was an example of the nanny-teacher assuming that the parents must be taught the rules of parenting. These rules are taught to parents for two reasons. The first reason is that the nanny wants to decrease her workload and make parents share some childcare responsibilities. The second reason (more often articulated in interviews) is that the nanny wants to create (what she sees as) better family relations and family environment for the child—and this she aims at achieving through teaching parents that daily physical contact is an essential part of their parenthood.

Teaching family activities was conditioned by the fact that room for manoeuver for families to do "family work" (or kin work; di Leonardo, 1987) was quite limited. As the children spend most of their active time with their nannies, parents have only evenings, nights and selected days to dedicate to "family time." Not only were the nannies very critical when it came to the *quantity* of time that parents spend with their children, they were also critical of the *qualitative* aspect of the activities. When describing the qualitative aspect of the family activities, the nannies framed them in the dichotomist ethnic framework of what *we* do (well) and what *they* do (wrong). The nannies complained that parents do not have time to go for a trip to visit a castle, which was for nannies a typical example and representation of how Czech families spend their leisure time à la Czech. It was quite commonly reported by both nannies and children that such activities were undertaken with the nannies, and not with parents (see Chapter 5). Framing the required family activities in ethnic terms, the nannies pointed out the advantages of their ethnic background in order to make their advice appear credible, heeded, and—above all—superior to anything the mothers do or do not. This enabled nannies to strengthen their respect and influence in the children's upbringing.

Lessons in care responsibilities usually go hand in hand with the previous two lessons. Nannies that formed emotional ties with the child in their care were willing to do anything for the cared-for children and their well-being. Nevertheless, they tried to maintain the limits of their responsibilities by refusing to perform some activities, and by teaching parents to do them. However, the nannies were then torn between satisfying the children's needs, and preserving some responsibilities as "mother-only." Such tension led them to try and teach mothers to take back some of their (wished-to-be-delegated) responsibilities—for example attending parent-teacher meetings at school. These lessons are taught in order to claim quantitative superiority in performing childcare tasks. As the list of tasks performed by mothers was shortened, and the list of tasks done by nannies was correspondingly lengthened, the nannies' knowledge about the children's lives became much greater than that of the parents. This fact served the nannies as an important source for this kind of moral hierarchy. If the two previous lessons were motivated by the qualitative superiority of nannies' care (the mothers should care in a *better* way), here the interviewees perceived themselves as "doing everything" for the children in their care, and accentuated their quantitative superiority (the mothers should care in a more *intensive* way).

And third, there were nannies who presented themselves as "boasting care-givers." Employing the last type of moral hierarchies, some nannies tended to minimize the parents' role in particular domains of the children's lives, and so present themselves as the children's primary care-giver. These nannies believe they have a far greater impact on the children's wellbeing and educational development than the children's own parents. While all the nannies called for recognition of their role in the child's life, the nannies that I label "boasting care-givers" did so at the expense of acknowledging the parents' role. "The mother cares about them, she works hard and we know she loves her children but … We have taught them everything," said Ms. Dudková. The interviews with "boasting care-givers" indicate the kind of moral hierarchies that are employed as a strategy to obtain recognition and praise for those aspects of their work which they most value. In all cases, a more or less explicit superiority over the mother is expressed when the nannies accentuate the aspects which only they (and not parents) can give the children at the moment—either because the parents are busy, or because they do not have the necessary skills (they do not speak Czech or do know "Czech activities" such as skiing, picking mushrooms, etc.).

To make their arguments about mothers' mothering and their own care-giving stronger, the nannies frame their criticism of Vietnamese mothers in ethnic terms. Using their "ethnic origin dividend" they present themselves as experts in mothering in the Czech Republic, and claim that mothers should (at least a little bit) follow what is represented as an ideal of mothering there. Being part of the majority—and hence aware of "how it goes here"—also means knowing how children should be brought up in the Czech Republic. Nannies declared themselves superior to Vietnamese mothers, whose customs they considered irrelevant to life in the Czech Republic. The nannies—as the possessors of a monopoly over knowledge of the "Czech way of raising children" in the employer-employee relationship—, use their ethnic background to gain advantage over the Vietnamese mothers. The logic of "they could/should do it if they want to live here" played an important role in ranking what the nannies saw as bad, good, and best motherhood strategies. At the same time, the nannies usually resort to ethnic explanations for the perceived failures in Vietnamese mothering. While the nannies are able to accommodate to Vietnamese children's physical otherness, they are unable to surmount the ethnic otherness of the mothers. This ethnic otherness also serves nannies as a ready explanation for the mothers "unacceptable" behavior toward their children: "Vietnamese mothers are just like that" or "Vietnamese mothers have it [unhealthy preference for work to family life] in their mentality" were common statements made by nannies, and formed part of the boundaries nannies drew between themselves and their employers, and between Czech mothering and Vietnamese mothering.

* * *

In summary, Czech nannies help Vietnamese mothers to enter the labour market. However, most nannies are convinced that the mother should stay home longer and/or that she should be more focused on her children. The nannies thus provide "a service in which they do not believe" (Nelson, 1994). The moral hierarchies play the role of defense mechanism, enabling the nannies to conceptualize the situation in which they find themselves when becoming nannies and—above all—to guard their ideals of good motherhood. As the establishment of moral hierarchies is built on their own understanding of motherhood, the extent to which the nannies accept *other* ways of mothering differs. The level of acceptance varied from total rejection (and the statement that "Vietnamese mothers are bad mothers") to partial understanding ("Vietnamese mothers are good mothers; however, they should …") to defense of the Vietnamese mothers' mothering strategies ("they are good mothers, they do what their conditions allow them to do"). Contrary to the mothers' conceptions of mothering, however, the nannies insist that mother must be the only (for nannies with the experience of full-time mothering) or at least primary (for previously working mothers) care-giver in the child's life, and breadwinning does not count as fulfilling mothering responsibilities.

4.3 Between Vietnamese Mother and Czech Nanny: Inter-generational Gaps and Reconciliations

How do children of Vietnamese immigrant parents who are brought up by Czech nannies think about care, family relations, and mothering? How do they perceive the differences between their ties with mothers and nannies and the differences in mothers' mothering and nannies' care-giving? The differences between a "Czech upbringing" and a "Vietnamese upbringing" became one of the main topics in the interviews and usually this issue was verbalized by children themselves without my asking. "I was lucky that my parents were not the typical Vietnamese parents," began many of child interviewees when describing the time spent with nanny and with parents. Bui, a 20-year-old girl, for instance continued: "My parents really wanted to spend time with me so they came to pick me up even if it was 10 pm so that I could sleep under one roof with them." Tuyet, a 21-year-old girl, said that she was very lucky because "my parents are now thinking more like Europeans, not Vietnamese." These statements contrast with the statements of several of children I interviewed who told me "My parents are like other Vietnamese, they focus only on working." Considering the different standpoints of my interviewees, I distinguish three categories of children according to how they perceive their mothers' mothering (and parents' parenting generally). They are: *complaining children* whose account was pervaded with stories about the unbridgeable distance between parents and child; *teaching children* who emphasized their influence on the parents' care-giving strategies; and *understanding* children who built their account around the main argument that "my parents did all this for me." Each of these categories portrays from different perspectives the active role of children in making sense of the institution of motherhood and childhood (what they mean, how motherhood should be performed), and of family in general (how family ties are defined).

4.3.1 Complaining Children: "We Don't Understand Each Other"

Thi, a 22-year-old girl, was born in Vietnam and came to the Czech Republic at the age of 5. Soon after their arrival, the parents started looking for a nanny with whom Thi could live until they earned some money and found a better apartment. She started living with her nanny; meanwhile the parents put all their efforts into running their business on the German-Czech border. They met with their daughter only on weekends, which destabilized their parent-child relations. Thi recalled this part of her childhood and its outcomes in the following words:

> At the beginning I did not want to go there [to her nanny] because I was very fixed on my mum. But then I very quickly got used to it. I got used to the fact that I go to Czech school, with Czech kids, that I am learning the Czech language. And I started breaking with our [Vietnamese] habits. Because I went home only for weekends and did not speak with my parents very much, I started forgetting Vietnamese. (…) And the relationship with my parents was weird. I liked them very much but at the same time I had no shared memories with them for those seven years when I was living in a Czech family. Thus at first I had to adjust to the Vietnamese regime, which was not a big problem. The biggest problem was the Vietnamese language. Fortunately, my dad speaks Czech so it was not a problem to talk with him. But with my mum, that was much worse at the beginning. And it prevails even now. I cannot speak with my mum because of the language barrier. (…) I think that my parents did not expect that I would forget Vietnamese so quickly and that I would adopt the Czech mentality so quickly. In recent years they have come to realize that I feel more like a Czech, and they know I will stay here when they go back to Vietnam. (…) Well because I lived in a Czech family, I do not have a close relationship with my parents. Not as close as I would wish. But I see how much my parents do for me and I admire them and appreciate it. I have a super relationship with them but it could be much better. We could be much closer to each other.

As in the story of Linh at the beginning of this chapter, Thi describes her ties with her parents as "not as close as she wishes." Her relationship with them is based on admiration and respect which, however, does not make the ties any warmer. There are many manifestations of the distance between parent and child, both having the same source: the lack of physical contact between children and parents and the intensive contact with a nanny who does not share the same ethnic background with the child. Apparently, not all of the children I interviewed experience this distance with the same intensity. A very simplistic equation works here: the less frequent the contact with parents (as in the case of live-in children), and the longer the time separated from the parents, the more distant the relationship during the period when mothering is delegated to nanny. What does this "distance" mean? There are three kinds of distances that the children mentioned extensively in the interviews: emotional distance, linguistic distance and mental distance.

When describing *emotional distance* and the ties with their parents, the children usually relied on an idealized picture of Czech families in which harmonious and warm ties are supposedly the norm, and which can never be found in Vietnamese families. The children paint this picture of supposed emotional closeness between members of Czech families on the basis of several sources: public discourse (such as movies, magazines, etc.), observations of their friends, their own experiences in Czech families, or simply as the opposite of what they observed in their own family. As the case of Linh shows:

> When I lived with my grandma and grandpa [nanny and her husband], they kept on showing me their love, they were hugging me, kissing me, and telling me how great I am and how much they love me. I guess it is like that in the Czech families. But Vietnamese are not like that at all. All the time they put me down, giving me examples of good Vietnamese children who were successful, they criticized me—all this in order to motivate me.

There are two essential elements in this account which shed light on how children may perceive the impact of delegated care, and the physical distance between them and the parents during childhood, on their current emotional ties with parents. First is Linh's interpretation of the parents' "emotion-giving." Like other interviewees, Linh frames the emotional distance between her and her parents in the dichotomy "Czech families" versus "Vietnamese families." Likewise Hanh, an 18-year-old girl, contrasted her perception of the parent-child ties in Czech families with those in Vietnam/Vietnamese families: "There parents must be respected, and parents when they have problems they just whisper it between them because it's not the child's business." In many other interviews the children referred to *respect* as the basis for their relationship with their parents, contrasting it with *emotions* which they considered a more appropriate and natural component of parent-child ties. This does not mean that the children did not love their parents; it only means that their love for their parents was based on respect, and not on the emotions and closeness they connected with "typical Czech families" and/or the families of their nannies.

Second is the understanding of emotional ties as the basis for parent-child ties. In all interviews, the delegation of care-giving was perceived as something that (temporarily) undermines the emotional closeness of the members of the family and it can even lead to questioning of the family ties themselves. As noted in the introductory story, Linh lived with her nanny until she was 10. Then she had to move to her parents, which she described as a huge change in her life. Since then, the 20-year-old interviewee told me, she has been trying to find her way back to her parents, but does not consider this effort as successful, relating that "I did not regard them as my parents, and they did not consider me their child." In her account, emotional closeness serves as the outcome, mark and confirmation of parenting, which must be performed in order that emotional ties be established, parents become parents, and the child becomes the parents' child.

The lack of physical contact shapes the *linguistic distance* between parents who speak Vietnamese and children who are brought up by Czech nannies in an environment where Czech is spoken. The language barrier between parents and children apparently goes hand in hand with emotional distance: children and parents cannot get closer to one another because they lack the tools to open up channels of communication. Because they are not close enough to each other, they have no need to communicate with each other, as they rarely have common topics for discussion. The importance of the Vietnamese language in the children's life was apparent in all interviews—not only because it was the only linguistic tool they could use for communicating with parents, but also because it was the marker of their "Vietnameseness," their ethnic identity. All children in my sample marked Vietnamese as their *mother* tongue. However, all of them also noted that they speak better Czech or even English than Vietnamese. It was their *nanny's* tongue in which they felt more comfortable and sure of themselves, and in which many of them said their first words. Minh, a 17-year-old boy, started attending language school and at the age of 17 began studying Vietnamese because he had difficulties keeping in touch with relatives in Vietnam. He did not speak Vietnamese at all: being a live-in child, his mother tongue was his nanny's mother tongue. Very often the Vietnamese language was learnt backwards, typically as a reaction to the emerging question of belonging and finding one's roots.

Language distance also impacts mutual understanding (comprehension) between parents and children—and produces intergenerational *mental distance*. Those children who did not speak Vietnamese well pointed out that a lack of shared vocabulary and conversation lead to a lack of common topics. In the children's view, language operates as a tool for transmitting what they called "mentality." In other words, language distance produces *mental distance*. When they say "we don't understand each other," children are not referring only to linguistic understanding, but also to understanding in the sense of sharing the same opinions, perspectives and worldviews. For many children, therefore, it is usually the nanny who is trusted and to whom the children confide, not the parents. This is so not only because they spend more time with their nannies than with their parents, but because their upbringing in a Czech family causes the children to feel mentally closer to their Czech nannies than to their Vietnamese parents.

4.3.2 Teaching Children: "You Must Bring Your Parents Up"

In the previous section I focused on the situation where nannies teach mothers lessons about mothering. Children also employed a similar practice towards their parents in their effort to get closer to their parents and develop emotional ties with them. The accounts make clear that children are able to both distinguish between childcare strategies (these experienced with nannies and those with parents), as well as sort and validate those strategies (in a similar way as the nannies formulate their moral hierarchies), and impose them on their parents. There were two lessons in particular that children sought to teach their parents: the lesson in physical contact, and the lesson in the philosophy of upbringing.

Physical contact and the parent-child relationship

I have already mentioned that some children in my sample started their stories about their parents with the statement that "Luckily, my parents are not typical Vietnamese." Employing the rhetoric of "luckiness" points to two significant issues in the parent-child relationship. First, children are aware that a childcare model exists within the Vietnamese community ("typical Vietnamese do this and that"), and they find this model inappropriate or even bad because of the lack of physical contact. The children stating that "*luckily* their parents are not typical Vietnamese parents" creates hierarchies of care-giving which are based on the sufficiency or lack of physical contact between children and parents. Thinking within such hierarchical rankings, the children rarely take into account the parenting/childcare models which are relevant in Vietnam (as discussed in Chapter 2). Instead, it is the parenting and childcare patterns they observe around them (friends, schoolmates, nanny's family, etc.) which have most relevance for them. Second, the children also reflect the position of their parents on the hierarchical scale of childcare models. As their comments suggest, they create in their imagination a continuum stretching from good parental care-giving to bad parental care-giving. Several child interviewees place their parents' model on the bad end of the spectrum—though their parents are "luckily" not *that* bad. However, there is a hidden point in these statements which plays a significant role in children's understanding of their parents' role: their parents do not approach the range of what the children consider a "good childcare model." In other words, the parents are "not as bad as typical Vietnamese parents," however, the way they perform childcare is "not as good as typical Czech parents." The quotation from the interview with Khanh, a 21-year-old university student, exemplifies the children's efforts to change the quantity and quality of time spent with parents, and by so doing, bridge or at least lessen the intergenerational and cultural gap between them.

> Adéla: Why did your parents close their business?
>
> Khanh: There were two reasons for this. First, the shop did not earn much. They were there all the time but without profit. And second, it was because of me and my younger sister. I remember I was at grammar school and the children around me talked about holidays, where they were going, and that their mums are with them during the weekend. I know it is my fault because I blame them for not being with us, they do not spend time with us. (…) I was crying so much that my sis does not have any childhood with them; she has no memories with them,

> except being with them at the market. And one month later my mum told me that she closed the business and will start working normally.

Khanh, as well as other children, accentuated in the interviews that the parents did all they could for them, and that the lack of physical contact was the "by-product" of the parents' effort to ensure a better future for their children. However, what this example shows in particular is the child's role in changing the parents' parenting and elevating it to a level that the children consider acceptable. Witnesses of children who persuaded their parents to modify their work in order save their relationship provide us with insight into how children may perceive delegated care-giving, and their ties with working parents. Above all, they illuminate the essential role of children in childcare negotiations, and the strength of their influence on parents' employment decisions as well as their philosophy of upbringing.

Parents' philosophy of upbringing and the children as teachers

Besides reporting that they were lucky that their parents spent more time with them compared to other Vietnamese parents, the children also reported another side of "luckiness." The children described how lucky they were that their parents were "not so conservative, and quite open to the European lifestyle." What does this mean exactly? The fact that the children I interviewed were between the ages of 16–25 years has impacted on how they talked about childrearing, and what aspects of their own upbringing they articulated as important. Very often it was the issue of the teenage life—such as their love life—which was most important for these children, and in which they demanded liberties that most Vietnamese parents usually refuse to grant their children. Many interviewees recalled how they used to be angry with their parents for not letting them to go to the pub with their schoolmates or friends. "While my Czech friends could be at the pub till midnight, I had to be home in the evening," was frequently repeated in the interviews. The children described their parents as too strict and conservative—for example when it came to their children's partner/love life. The children I interviewed often described that their parents as being against unmarried cohabitation and dating at an early age.

When recollecting the parents' attitudes towards her and her upbringing, Tuyet told a story about how she quarreled with her father about who she was and where she belonged. "I said in front of my parents that I am Czech and my dad got really angry with me," as Tuyet described an incident that happened when she was around 15 years old. "And my dad began explaining to me that I am not Czech, I cannot be Czech because I have Vietnamese parents so I am Vietnamese." Recalling this talk, Tuyet started explaining her influence on her parents which helped them to overcome the distance between them. She described to me how her father could not understand her, and she was forced to explain to him that she was brought up in Europe and that her "mentality" (to use her word) was European. "It was hard, but I educated my parents. Now my parents understand me because I educated them." Tuyet offered a couple of examples, including her parents' openness to her love life, to prove the results of her teaching. Such teaching meant the slight shift in her parents' mentality—the shift from conservative Asian attitudes to more lenient, European ones.

4.3.1 Understanding Children: "They Did It for Me"

The argument embedded in the title of this section was echoed in many interviews, as it provided children (even the complaining ones) with a step towards reconciling their relations with their parents. At the same time, in the accounts it usually played the role of demonstrating the child's maturation and deep changes in his/her understanding of ethnic identity, position in the family, and belonging. As in Bui's account, when she describes the transformation of her attitudes from childhood to adulthood:

> When I was younger, I liked the Czech way of upbringing because it is less strict. My parents did not let me go anywhere because they were afraid for me. But the older I get, the more I understand them, and I am coming closer to the Vietnamese again. Because before, I had turned away from them.

Bui's account highlights that mutual understanding between parents and children is something which does not necessarily exist, but which is developed and achieved when the child turns back to his or her parents and Vietnamese roots. Contrary to what was described by Khanh or Tuyet, who, decided to change their parents, Bui changes her understanding of the situation, and starts returning to her parents.

Even though the children express their regret about not being able to spend more time with their parents, they emphasized that their parents have given up everything for their children to have a better life in Europe. For parents, being in the Czech Republic *for* their children also meant being *without* their children. Part of what parents had to give up was their family life. When several of my interviewees stated, "They gave up their family life so that I could have my family life with nanny," they were pointing out a basic element of their mothers' mothering: a good mother provides her children with the best, giving them as many opportunities and life chances as possible. Here again, the issue of respect and gratitude of children towards their parents becomes the leitmotif of parent-child ties, which are understandably interpreted within the post-migratory challenges to family life. All in all, these children—usually when adult, and looking back—adopted their mothers' definition of motherhood: a role that is carried out primarily in the labour market through breadwinning activity.

* * *

The generation gap (as perceived by children) crystallizes around the emotional, linguistic, and mental distance between children and parents, and is the unintended consequence of the delegation of mothering. It is unintended and surprising to parents, who expected their children to remain their children, to remain Vietnamese, to speak Vietnamese, and to have a Vietnamese mentality. Children described their parents as relying on pre-existing child-parent ties, which exist simply because the parents are the parents and the children are their children. This chimes with my interviews with the mothers, who were not afraid of losing touch with their children when sending them to nannies, and often argued that "children know who their parents are." Contrary to such a primordial definition of parent-child ties, the children stressed the necessity of developing and reinforcing parent-child ties in order to perform and maintain what the parents consider a "given" relationship. That is why children interpreted this generational and cultural gap as the logical consequence of having been brought up in by Czech nannies, who provided the children with emotional ties as well as social and cultural capital transmission. In the children's perspective, a language must be spoken in order to not be forgotten, and must be spoken with parents in order to not drift away from one's parents, and in order to continue to understand one another.

Observing the emergence of the generational gap, the children take various positions—some of them complain, some of them successfully try to change it, and some of them accept it as an inevitable consequence of living in Europe and appreciate their parents' self-sacrifice in the labour market. Their accounts clearly show the active role of children in childcare negotiations, particularly in the cases where children present themselves as their parents' teachers. In this section, it became clear that the children are not only a passive—car*ed for*—link in the relationship with active—car*ing*—mothers and nannies. The children reflect their parents' parenthood, make sense of it, and actively intervene in their parents' childcare styles. These children enjoy a strong position in family life negotiations, and hence shape their own childcare in ways they consider best for themselves.

4.4 Provisional Conclusions: Children Growing Up and Becoming Responsible

When delegating motherhood, Vietnamese immigrant mothers simulate the model of childcare common in Vietnam in order to provide their children with living conditions that enable the children to overcome the migration status of their parents and to integrate into Czech society. However, the parents' efforts are rarely appreciated by the nannies, or by the children themselves until they reach adult age. For nannies and for children, the Vietnamese parent/entrepreneur becomes a symbol of both diligence and bad parenthood. On the one hand Vietnamese parents are hard-working and self-sacrificing, who do all that they can to provide a better future for their children by earning money. On the other hand, the Vietnamese parents do not spend much time with their children; they delegate childcare responsibilities to other women; and—in the vocabulary of nannies and children—prefer work to care-giving. Nevertheless, the delegation of motherhood from immigrant mothers to native nannies shapes the mothers,' nannies' and children's understanding of motherhood and care-giving. It impacts how childhood is constructed and experienced by second generation Vietnamese children, and what the conditions for integration are for Vietnamese first generation Vietnamese mothers. The testimony of Quyen, a 21-year-old girl living in the Czech Republic since the age of 6, portrays the consequences of motherhood delegation:

> I think that most Vietnamese parents, they send their children to Czech families not only because they want their kids to learn the language, but so the children are later able to help them, their parents, with the Czech language, the Czech community, and just to understand the problems that they do not understand very well (like law, education, the economy, contracts and administrative issues, etc.). And they do not think about the consequences, that their children will forget how to speak Vietnamese. When my dad gave me a contract, I understood it but I could not explain it in Vietnamese. So they started reproaching me that I attend school and I cannot explain it. They didn't think I would forget Vietnamese.

The account of Quyen, as well as other interviewees, makes evident that motherhood delegation brings the three-fold mutual transmission of responsibilities and skills between mothers, nannies, and children. This transmission proceeds in three steps which are illustrated in Figure 4.1.

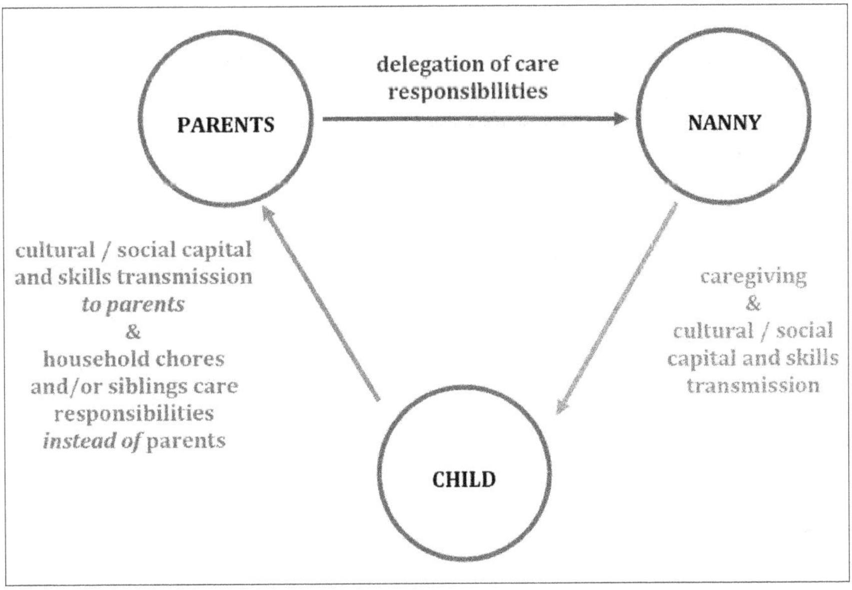

Figure 4.1 Three-fold mutual transmission of responsibilities and skills between mothers, nannies, and children

The first step in the three-fold delegation entails the delegation of childcare responsibilities from mothers/parents to nanny. This chapter demonstrates that the nannies become responsible for satisfying the children's basic needs, for transmitting skills, social and cultural capital, and to a certain extent making decisions about the child. The second step is the result of the everyday tasks of care-giving, where care-givers pass care-giving to care receivers. When childcare is delegated from mothers to nannies, the nannies also take on other tasks—sometimes directly connected to the cared-for child (doctor or school visits), or sometimes related to other family members (such as helping parents with administrative necessities, insurance, etc.). Doing all these things, the nanny slowly initiates children into these responsibilities, and later it is the child who starts playing the crucial role in dealing with institutions outside the household. Thus the nanny—through her care-giving—, directly passes cultural and social capital and skills to the children, and indirectly delegates to the children responsibilities that she received from the children's parents.

And finally, the third step represents 1) the transmission of skills taught by nannies from children to parents; and 2) the performance by children of household chores and/or care-giving of younger siblings. The termination of a nanny's paid care-giving does not imply that the mother returns to the household nor that household chores or care-giving of younger siblings disappear. Rather it is now up to the older children to take on these responsibilities. As evident in Linh's story at the beginning of this chapter, when children are somewhat older (usually at about 13) they are expected to start helping parents with family tasks—household chores, communication with institutions outside the household (Kibria, 1993), or helping parents in their businesses (see Song, 1999). Thanks to their language competencies and social skills, the children become interpreters and mediators between parents and mainstream society, often acting as "representatives" of their parents in performing activities normally reserved for the adult parents, such as communicating with bureaucracies.

There are two consequences of this delegation that illuminate the specificity of family ties, family division of labour, and integration of family members in Vietnamese families in relation to the findings of the existing scholarship.

First, the experiences of immigrant families with delegated mothering radically differ from the experiences of immigrant families that do not delegate childcare to nannies. The model in which second generation children, thanks to their language knowledge, become mediators between family and outside institutions has been described in other studies (Kibria, 1993; Guo, 2014; Orellana, Dorner and Pulido, 2003). These studies also demonstrate the importance of "bridging activities" in "settling" *first* generation immigrants, especially mothers. Bridging activities include communication with bureaucracies, schools, incorporation into the local neighborhood, etc., and are normally performed by women in the country of origin. In the host country, however, these activities take on a new dimension (Kibria, 1993; Ryan, 2007). They become the means of integrating immigrant mothers, and establishing social capital and skills that help these women adapt to the new country. In the case of Vietnamese families, however, delegation of mothering also means delegation of "bridging activities," and offers parents (mothers) the option *not* to participate in those activities, and so and thus *not* to integrate into mainstream society. As these bridging activities are performed first by nannies and then by children, nannies and children serve as mediators between parents and the host culture, and allow parents to not invest their time in anything else but their business (integration competences are no exception). With their sights set on a future return to Vietnam, an intensive working life within the immigrant economy leaves no time for gaining other skills than those needed in the shop or business.

A second important point must be made in regard to the scholarship on care work. This brings us back to Joan C. Tronto and her article on the nanny question in feminism (Tronto, 2002). "What is the consequence for children of growing up with another adult charged with their care?" Tronto asks (*ibid.*, p.40) and her answer is the following: "Children may well come to expect that other people, regardless of their connection to them, will always be available to meet their needs. They may come to treat people as merely means, and not as ends in themselves." Interviews with children with experience of being brought up by nannies indicate a rather different conclusion. First, far from treating their nannies as "merely means," the children develop deep emotional and kinship ties with them (Chapter 5). Second, if children have any expectations about other people being available to meet their needs when they are small, this expectation very soon disappears, as it is usually superseded by the burden of assuming household responsibilities. Linh described her first day back at her parents' when her mother told her: "We go to work, we come back around 10 pm, so you must prepare lunch, iron the laundry, clean, and look after your 2-year-old-brother." The 13-year-old girl did not know how to do all this, but she quickly she realized that she would have to learn, as her brother was dependent on her, there simply was nobody else to do the household chores.

The children in my sample usually compared themselves to their schoolmates, recalling that they were not allowed to go out with them because they had to be home to perform domestic work. Likewise, nannies compared the abilities of Vietnamese children with their own children or with "typical Czech children." For instance, Ms. Andulková described the enormous autonomy of Anh, who at the age of 12 became responsible for the household. The nanny remarked that she could not imagine any Czech child doing as much as Anh did. These experiences contrast greatly with what Tronto (2002) suggested in her article. This is probably because of differences in the family backgrounds of Vietnamese families compared to the families analyzed in the mainstream scholarship that Tronto refers to. It may be that in the middle-class Western families that hire immigrant care workers, the behavior of children that Tronto described was prevalent. The analysis of the interviews with children and nannies clearly demonstrates that Vietnamese families are far from falling into this pattern.

In addition, the analysis also shows how childhood is defined. The children participate in the adult world, and help their parents navigate in the new world. When taking on these adult activities, children free their families from dependence on people outside the family. Such an understanding of childhood is not in conflict with children's performance of "adult" activities. On the contrary, the performance of these activities is an inevitable part of these children's post-migratory lives. As many studies show, this role assumed by second generation children is a common strategy of adaptation in the new society, and is a natural response to social and cultural changes brought on by migration (Guo, 2014). Nevertheless, this experience is even more pronounced when childcare and domestic tasks are delegated and parenthood is performed within the labour market. In addition, it must be added that in the case of Vietnamese immigrants, it is a strategy that reflects the definition of the migratory project as temporary, in which first generation immigrants feel no need to learn Czech and/or integrate into Czech society.

Chapter 5
"From Nanny to Granny": Caring as Kinning

> "And then he once told me: 'granny, I know you are not my own granny, but are we not lucky to have met?' He completely destroyed me by saying this."
>
> Ms. Havranová, nanny of Chien

My name is Minh Truong and I am 17 years old. Since I was born, I have been living with my mum in a small town. I was born in the Czech Republic—my mum came here in the 1990s. Here she met my father, but their relationship did not last very long so that is why I only live with her now. My mother used to work at a market place in the town center—in summer, winter; she was there all the time. Now she has her own shop, around 10 kilometers from here. So nowadays it is better; however, there are not enough clients these days.

When my mum was working at the outdoor market, she met my grandpa, Mr. Kos. Well, at that time he was not my grandpa of course. They started talking and they got along very well. Then my mum met Mr. Kos' wife, Ms. Kosová. Sometime later I was born, and when my mum and I were in the maternity hospital, Ms. and Mr. Kos came to see us and help my mum to solve some problems. After that, my mum wanted Ms. Kosová to become my nanny—I know it from my mother. However, she could not because she had her job and she had to work. When my mum was obliged to return to work at her shop, because we did not have enough money to survive, I started being looked after by a Czech woman. I was with her from Monday to Friday. Friday afternoons, after my nanny finished work, Ms. Kosová picked me up and I was with her over the weekend. And she was a much better nanny than the other woman. Then something great happened: Ms. Kosová had the opportunity to retire two years earlier than we had expected, and she immediately started taking care of me. Suddenly, I had a "granny."

After that I began living at my granny's. There I had my own room and toys and everything. It was a kind of an inheritance from my granny's children. I remember that I liked watching fairy tales on television. My granny had many TV channels; that was great. We did everything together. I liked cleaning the house with her: she did the vacuuming and me, I got the duster and ran around with it. That was a nice division of labour. My mum came to see me every day after work, just for a while because she was busy and very tired after work. I did not spend much time with her, which is why I now have a big problem with the Vietnamese language. I had to start attending language school. I cannot speak Vietnamese at all. When I talk with my grandfather in Vietnam, it is a huge problem. I do not understand him at all. My teacher once called grandma, and she had to come to my school and she was asked what that was supposed to mean. I was so confused, for me it was apparent that if my granny is Kosová, I must be Kos, too. Today we recall this story and laugh together. It is funny—I knew what her name was because I could see it everywhere—on the mailbox, on the door ring, and I also heard how she was addressed when we went somewhere together. And I somehow connect my surname with her and not with my mum.

When someone asks me what my relationship with grandma is, I answer without any hesitation that it is thanks to her that I know what I know and that I am who I am. If I had to write a list of reasons why she is so important for me, it would go:

1. Because she speaks Czech and she could teach me Czech more than my parents ever could.
2. Because she can prepare a Czech meal. If I had to eat only rice, I would be fed up soon. My mum can prepare a Czech meal, too, but my granny is better at it.
3. Because she had more time to be with me and she could focus intensively on me. For example, when I did not know something at school, she helped me. Now I do not need this because I have the internet; but before, she was my only advisor.
4. And finally, because I can say I have a grandmother. I always say I'm going to my grandma's, and people often wonder what my Vietnamese grandmother is doing here! They do not understand that she is my Czech granny.

* * *

Paid care-giving always generates emotional ties. These ties are conceptualized in everyday care-giving practice as kinship ties. However, only some of these emotional ties are actually *kinned*. What makes a kinned relationship possible between nanny, child, and parents? And what does kinning means for the three actors?

To answer the first question we must backtrack a bit in our discussion, and in the lives of both families and their nannies. In Chapter 2 and Chapter 3 I argued that the post-migratory reconstruction of immigrant family life (by the families), and the character of caring biographies and intergenerational relations (on the part of nannies) are the main sources of motivation to hire and or become a nanny. Inspired by Nazli Kibria (1993) and her research on the "family tightrope" and negotiations of generational and gendered relations in immigrant families, I argue that hiring a nanny is an inherent part of "unpacking the cultural baggage" that Vietnamese immigrants bring with them from Vietnam. According to my argument, nanny recruitment is an attempt on the part of Vietnamese families to recreate the traditional Vietnamese family model, which includes not only childcare but also emotional and practical support, and the feeling of being part of the social network. Simply put, the nannies are cast in the role that the grandmother traditionally plays in Vietnam. How this role is played out here in the Czech Republic is up to the nannies, the children, and their parents. As for the nannies, their caring biographies must again be addressed—and in particular the role of childcare in the nanny's life, and the nature of her inter-generational ties. In Chapter 3, I discussed how particular kinds of nannies' caring biographies supply the demands of Vietnamese families. The need to be needed, the need for intergenerational ties, and the importance of childcare for women's self-identity are critical factors in establishing emotional and kinship ties with cared children.

To understand the way ties between nannies and children (and less often parents) are established as kinship ties, I argue that caring should be understood as an essential part of the *kinning* process. I have borrowed this concept from Signe Howell (2003) whose contribution to contemporary kinship studies is undeniable. Based on a constructivist perspective on kinship, Howell's research on transnational adoption leads her to develop the concept of kinning as: "the process by which a foetus, new-born child (or *any previously unconnected person*) is brought into a significant and permanent relationship which is expressed in a kin idiom" (Howell, 2003, p. 465, italics added). This concept brings to light a new dimension in paid care relations and provides us a nuanced picture of kinship relations, and of the role of care-giving in establishing and maintaining kinship ties. Employing this concept, I trace the process of how the nanny becomes a granny, and how the cared-for child becomes a grandchild. I include in my study the parents of Vietnamese children and their grandparents living in Vietnam as well, in order to shed greater light on the process of establishing and maintaining kinship ties through daily care-giving, and a sense of family belonging. In Chapter 6 I continue this discussion, dealing with how a sense of belonging is created, transmitted and negotiated through the account/experience of kinship. There I focus on how the language of kinship and of belonging *intra-act*, by which I mean how they influence and overlap one another to shape an entwined sense of belonging. The two chapters address children's perceptions of their belonging to kinship and to national homeland both of which balance between references to biogenetic and social relatedness. In doing so, they illuminate how children make sense of their belonging in relation to care-giving and kinship ties.

As is evident from the title of this chapter, I examine care as an essential part of kinning. In section 5.1 I elaborate possible interpretations of kinship terminology, while in section 5.2 I examine three activities—addressed in interviews with children and nannies—that are critical to establishing kinship ties. These activities are: parent-responsibility substitute activities, family ritual activities, and exclusive (Czech) grandma activities. An examination of these activities sheds light on the daily negotiations of being a member of the family; on the connectedness of nannies with their children, grandchildren, and Vietnamese children; and finally on the relationships between my Vietnamese child interviewees and their Czech and Vietnamese grandmothers.

5.1 Grandma, Bà and Babi: Three Stories of One Word

When recruiting my potential interviewees, I asked them a seemingly simple question: "Did you ever have a Czech woman who took care of you?" They answered: "Yes, I have had a Czech grandma." Or "Yes, I have had a Czech aunt." Their answers revealed that my question was not only not simple, but that, above all, did not follow the *emic* perspective of interviewees.

There are three possible interpretations for using the words "grandma," and/or "aunt" and for using kinship terminology, in general. One linguistic interpretation suggests that employment of the word "grandma" or "aunt" does not refer to kinship terminology, but rather to the relative age of the nanny. A second interpretation—symbolic in nature—sees kinship terminology as a way to make sense of the relationship within delegated childcare, but without assuming established kinship ties. And finally a third interpretation considers the performative meaning of kinship terms, which is central to the argument that care establishes kinship ties. In this section I will look at each of these interpretations to explain my analytical approach in this chapter, and to briefly uncover the various statuses of kinship terminology and its place in the nanny-child relationship.

First there is the interpretation of the *linguistic meaning*—the semantics—of the word "grandma" in the Vietnamese language. The basic usage of the word "grandma" must be sought within the logic of the Vietnamese language. The word "bà" in Vietnamesee ("grandmother/grandma" in English) designates the kinship term "grandmother"—both one's mother's mother (*bà ngoại* where *ngoại* refers to grandmother on the *mother's* side) and one's father's mother (*bà nội* where *nội* refers to grandmother on the *father's* side), respectively. However, the word "bà" is also used to refer to any woman of similar age to one's own grandmother. The same is true for the word "cô"—which is equivalent to the word "aunt" in English—but which is also used to designate women of similar age to one's mother. Hence, addressing the nanny as "bà" or "cô" is not necessarily employing kinship terminology, but meant rather to refer to the relative seniority or status of the care-giver in question. Depending on the speaker, "bà" and "cô" may merely be a polite way of referring to any woman—similar to the word "lady" in English. In summary, the answer to the question "Why do Vietnamese children call their nannies grandmothers or aunts?" would be that the words "grandma"/"aunt" are used not as a denotation of kinship, but simply connote the word "lady."

The second interpretation considers the *symbolic meaning* of the kinship terminology in order to make sense of the nanny-child relationship. This understanding of kinship terminology usage refers to what the authors describe as "kinship-like," "pseudo-kinship" or "false kinship" ties between care-givers and the families they work for. From this point of view, kinship terminology provides a framework within which roles are defined. Using kinship terminology not only makes the relationship understandable within the intimate context of family life, but also establishes what the nanny can and should do with the child (Murray, 1998). Pei-Chia Lan (2002, p.187) argues that "a fictive kin relationship improves the quality of care and retrieves personal meanings for both the provider and the recipient." The role of the emotional ties that are awakened when the relationship is framed in symbolic terms such as "grandma" or "aunt" can play a dual role. On the one hand, these terms support and become a fundamental base for the kinning process, as will be discussed below.

On the other hand, however, they can be misused against nannies in the name of moral economy (for the abusive character of the rhetoric "one of the family" see Hess and Puckhaber, 2004; Anderson, 2000). Ms. Křepelková described her "kinship-like" role in the family by saying that "they take you as an aunt, but temporarily. When they stop needing you, you are not their aunt anymore." While Ms. Křepelková's experiences concur with the findings of the dominant research, this was generally not the case with the nannies in my study, perhaps because of the structure of my sample. Aside from a few exceptions, the overwhelming majority of nannies in my study did not experience "instrumental," temporary kinship ties. Acknowledging these cases, I want to avoid the romantic and idealistic notion that Vietnamese families' employment of Czech nannies always leading to symbiosis, and emotional and kinship ties. The process of kinning analyzed here does not occur automatically whenever a delegated childcare relationship is established. In the second interpretation, then, the word "grandma" relies on its denotative aspect—signifying, prescribing and making clear and simple the rules and roles within the relationship—but without any reference to the existence of kinship ties beyond these denotations.

The third interpretation—and the one of greatest relevance in this chapter—is that of *performative* meaning of kinship terminology. An illustrative example of the conceptualization of the relationship is the insight of Mai, a 17-year-old Vietnamese girl, who describes the issue of kinship categories and substance which was commonly mentioned in many interviews with children: "When I always say that I must go to my granny, my friends ask whether my grandmother from Vietnam is here. So I tell them then that she is a nanny. But it is strange for me to call my granny nanny. I feel such 'ah' [face contemptuously]." What Mai's account makes evident is the tension between two folk concepts (not just the words): the nanny and the grandma. For Mai, evidently, the word "grandma" is far from being just a designation or classification of pseudo-kinship relationships. Rather it reflects what Marshall Sahlins calls a "performative kinship" (Sahlins, 1985; 2011) between Mia and her nanny. Mia insists on calling her nanny "grandma," because to Mai, this woman *is her grandmother*. Stating that "whatever is construed genealogically may also be constructed socially" (Sahlins, 2011, p.3), Sahlins emphasizes the everyday maintenance and reproduction of post-natal kinship ties, and bases his argument on many anthropological studies on kinship. He is very much aware of the daily tasks of kinship that relatives must perform in order to be relatives: "The existing relations between persons are potentially unstable: continuously vulnerable to events and ever subject to negotiation" (*ibid.*, p.5).

These negotiations between nannies and cared-for children will be addressed in following section. Considering the relationship between nannies and children as part of performative kinship allows us to depict how "kinship is in this way the perduring condition of the possibility of its (unstable) practice" (*ibid.*, p.6). Such kinning practices (again using Howell's concept) results in kinship constellations where the nanny is addressed as grandma because she really *is* the child's grandma, and child is addressed as grandchild because he or she really *is* the nanny's grandchild.

5.2 Caring as Kinning: On Becoming Grandchild and Grandmother

In this section I focus on the issue of how Czech nannies become grandmothers and Vietnamese children become grandchildren. What kind of performative actions are necessary? Both nannies and children are part of their kinship networks: children in my sample are their parents' children, their grandparents' grandchildren, etc., while nannies in my sample are their children's mothers and, if they have any, their grandchildren's grandmothers. These ties are addressed in the interviews based on common genealogy and symbolized by biogenetic factors such as blood or genes. However, during the process of care-giving, kinship ties between cared-for children and caring nannies are established, maintained, and negotiated through the many daily practices that are emphasized in all the interviews. This section looks into the way family ties are re-negotiated through child care arrangements. Here I address the process of kinning by dealing with those aspects of the nanny-child relationship that both nannies and children in my sample marked as ties-establishing, and where they discussed the roles that are played on the basis of the kin idiom. The accounts about kinship are filled with the duality of what is the substance of kinship ties—whether they just *are*, or they are done—and as such they illuminate the ambivalence of belonging to the kinned trajectory, as well as belonging to the homeland (see Chapter 6).

Despite the diversity of both children's and nannies' experience, the accounts of what lies behind the formation of ties were surprisingly similar among my interviewees. The nannies and children enumerated many aspects of everyday life, all of which had a common denominator: intensive physical contact and shared memories. In what follows I will examine three kinds of activities that were significant for children's understanding of the role of the grandma in their lives and *vice versa*. These activities are: (1) parents'-responsibility substitute activities; (2) family ritual activities; and (3) exclusive (Czech) grandma activities. Classifying these activities into three groups is useful for illustrating the distinct ontological nature of these activities in the context of family life, parent-nanny sharing of childcare, and children's understanding of the nature of kinship ties with Czech and Vietnamese grandmothers. It is important to note that all interviewees whose stories are presented in this section exemplify the enduring nature of these ties: the Czech grandmothers (both nanny-interviewees and nannies of child interviewees) were—at the moment of conducting the interview—no longer providing paid care-giving services, yet still considered themselves "grandmothers" of the children they had taken care of.

5.2.1 Package One: Parents-Responsibility Substitute Activities

The first set of activities can be labelled as "parents'-responsibility substitute activities." This category encompasses activities which are performed by a grandmother because she is the primary care-giver. The nannies in my sample were recruited for very distinct tasks performed within very distinct timetables for children of very distinct ages. On one end of the age continuum there are children whose care by a nanny started when they were a few months old; on the other are children who had their first nanny when they started attending elementary school. Timetables of care consequently varied between 24 hours a day/7 days a week, to 4 hours a day/5 days a week. From this, it is already apparent that in many cases there is a vast quantitative and qualitative discrepancy between the time children spend with their nannies and the time they spend with their parents. The common dilemma that families recruiting nannies face is the disproportion of so-called "quality time" that children spend with their nannies, as opposed to with their parents.

Almost all of my child interviewees described their time spent with nanny as "active" time—filled with many activities such as games, trips, and learning—while time spent with parents was usually referred to as "passive" or even "no" time. When talking about her grandmother, I asked 16-year-old Mia whether she could imagine her life without her grandma, and what would be different. Without hesitating she told me: "I think I would have been alone most of the time; the parents had to be at work. And if I hadn't been with grandma, I would have simply been alone." Another frequent comment among child interviewees recalling their early childhood was: "My granny taught me everything." The influence of parents is temporarily sidelined, and the nanny becomes central to the life of child—the person who is always there for a child to listen, help, and give advice, and with whom the relationship is composed of intimacy, trust and spontaneously-generated emotion. Both for children and nannies, the large amount of time spent together was the most appreciated aspect of their relationship, as it created the basic "substance" of their kinship ties—*shared memories.* The case study of Khanh and Ms. Orlová illustrates it.

5.2.1.1 Khanh: "with grandma or alone"

Khanh was four years old when she came to the Czech Republic with her parents. They first lived in an area inhabited mainly by Vietnamese, and her parents ran a business on the German-Czech border. When Khanh began attending kindergarten, one of her teachers, Jindřiška Valová, became Khanh's nanny, after much persuasion by the parents. Khanh spent time at kindergarten with other children, and in the afternoons and weekends she was with her nanny, who soon became her "grandma." A two-hour-long interview with Hanh—now a 21-year old university student—revealed many common features of the role of care-giving in creating kinship ties. These are: *mutual trust and responsibility between grandmother and grandchild; the creation of shared memories; the establishment of a strong grandma-grandchild unit; and the imagined inclusion of the child in the grandmother's kin trajectory*. Before looking at each of these aspects, I will let Khanh explain who is a grandmother to her, what grandmothering means to her, and how she sees the role of the grandmother in her life.

> When you say "grandma," it is first and foremost my Czech grandma who comes into my mind. When I close my eyes I can see her. But I know somewhere deep inside myself that I have grandmas in Vietnam. And with the word "grandma" I image the person I have always wanted—someone with whom you can talk about your problems and who does a lot of things with you that parents cannot do because they are busy.

The children's accounts—including Khanh's—make clear that (at least in a particular period of life) the nanny becomes the person who knows the child best and whom the child trusts most. A number of my interviewees turned to their grandmothers when they needed to confide something, seek advice, or to just chat. Often this was because the nannies were physically present—while the parents, by contrast, were usually busy working or tired—or because the children were more linguistically competent in Czech than in Vietnamese, and so found it easier and more natural to speak in Czech to their nannies rather than in Vietnamese to the parents. While this was not the case with Khanh—who is fluent in Vietnamese—many children reported that they could not confide their problems to their parents because they did not "speak the same language." Whatever the reason—busy parents or language barriers—the grandmother almost always becomes the main trusted and listening ear, and the one that encourages and helps the child with his or her problems. Obviously, the mutual trust between grandma and grandchild does not "just" exist, but is achieved through mundane daily rituals and practices, such as asking the child how his day went when he comes back from school. Channels of communication are much more established with grandmas than with parents, as it is normally the grandma rather than the parents who is always there and ready to listen. In the evening when the parents come to pick up the child, whatever problems the child has have either already been solved or made less urgent, thanks to the grandmother's intervention earlier in the day.

As the child spends most of his or her "active time" with the nanny, it is the nanny who is mainly responsible for the child's daily care. This includes ensuring not only the child's physical wellbeing, but also his or her proper conduct and moral training. Apparently, such extensive responsibility on the part of the nanny towards the child is nothing surprising, and is a common feature in all relationships of delegated childcare (Nelson, 1994; Macdonald, 2010). However, Khanh's account indicates that there is a *mutuality* of responsibility which transcends the general understanding of responsibility in the nanny-child relationship (broadly defined as trust in the nanny's abilities to provide for the child). Of the many stories Khanh told me during the interview, two of those stories were particularly significant for her. Both stories provide us with insight into how mutual responsibility is established on a daily basis, and how building this mutuality is an essential part of the kinning process. The first story takes us back to Khanh's childhood, when she spent time with her grandmother doing many activities, such as taking walks. During one of these walks, the following incident happened:

> Once we were walking somewhere and I fell into a dunghill. Grandma told me not to go there, but I did, and I slipped right there. And I was too afraid to tell her because I had this guilty feeling—you know the feeling a granddaughter has for her granny. So I tried to fix it, wipe it off, but it smelt so much. So I had to tell her what had happened. And you know what? She spanked me and I cried (…) She was my granny "all inclusive," she was not like some women who don't dare raise their hand against a child. She took me as her granddaughter, so that when I am naughty, I simply had to be spanked.

The moral duty Khanh articulates here demanded that she "not disappoint" her grandmother. Her feelings of guilt were the outcome of not obeying her grandmother and making her sad. This is interpreted by her as the "feeling which the granddaughter has." She wishes to not disappoint her grandma not because she would be afraid of being punished, but because their relationship requires mutual responsibility, regard for one another, and respect for the emotional investment the grandmother has made in her. At the same time, Khanh's account reveals her appreciation toward her grandma for taking full responsibility over her upbringing. By accepting her punishment, and crediting it as a sign of her nanny's genuine love for her, Khanh truly sees her nanny, Ms. Valová, as her grandmother, with whom she has a true and deep relationship.

The second story took place during the holiday when Khanh was spending time with her nanny's grandchildren. Khanh had a very nice relationship with her nanny's granddaughter, but not with her grandson. One day Khanh and the grandson were playing together, and the boy wanted her to say "Tachov" (the name of a particular town) backwards. Though Khanh did not want to say it, the grandson insisted so strongly that she finally conceded and said—"vohcat" ("to screw," in English). In the end Khanh found the joke very funny and laughed. The following day Khanh was sitting at the table and eating lunch with her nanny's family, when she said to her grandpa (her nanny's husband), "Say Tachov backwards!." When the grandfather did, her grandma immediately froze in anger, and asked Khanh "Who told you this? You cannot say that word! It is very rude!" Khanh started to cry, and told her that it was Pája, her grandson, who had told her. Ms. Valová then began arguing with her daughter, telling her that she should teach her son manners, and that she, Ms. Valová, did not want her grandson teaching Khanh such things. "Aunt Jana (the nanny's daughter) was so angry with me," recalled Khanh, and refused to speak to either Khanh or her mother. "And I felt so guilty and I knew I should have never have told her about Pája. And she [the nanny] had turned against her daughter to protect me." Enjoying protection from grandma had meant grandma's turning against her own family—an event of great importance to Khanh, as it *really* proved the depth of her ties with her grandmother.

These stories shed light on how kinship ties are established in everyday activities, and how shared memories serve to maintain feelings of belonging, and of forming part of a single network of family relations. These stories are important not only because they were actually experienced and played an essential role in the kinning process, but also because they are transformed into shared memories that further strengthen already-established relations. In many interviews, the description and account of childhood centered around the grandmother. It seems that the grandmother was for most interviewees *the epitome of childhood*; the time spent with her was described as active and filled with many events which shaped a relationship based on mutual trust and mutual responsibility. This contrasted with the image of childhood spent without the grandmother, and with only the parents; "without granny I would be alone, or with my parents in the market place." When evoking the role of parents in their childhood, the interviewees usually stated that "the parents were too tired when coming home from work" or "they had no energy for doing anything together." The children understood this, even though some of them felt sorry for not being able to spend more time with their parents. The daily activities carried out with grandmothers were even more valued by children, as they were seen—besides the time spent with friends or schoolmates—as the *only* real quality time of their day.

This intensive daily contact creates (temporally) the inseparable unit of the grandma-granddaughter. "Wherever I went, I went there with my grandma," Khanh told me, and added that wherever her grandma went, everybody expected that she would go with her. Public recognition of the pair "grandma-child" plays an important role in both the child's and the nanny's self-presentation to people around them. Being kinned as a grandchild of a Czech grandmother, and conversely, as a grandmother of a Vietnamese grandchild, personhood is qualified through their relations to one another (see Howell, 2003). When Khanh says "I was visiting her friends with her," she is noting a significant outcome of her intensive contact with grandma who mediated her inclusion into networks not only based on friendship, but also on kinship. Neither nanny, child, nor the nanny-child unit are islands; the nannies are part of the children's kinship network (as mothers and grandmothers) and the children are part of the nannies' network (as children and grandchildren). The question that emerges here is: In which of these two kinship networks will the newly established unit of grandma-grandchild be placed—in the children's or in the nannies'? In other words, whose kinship network becomes the main point of reference? The majority of cases in my sample suggest that the most widespread model is where the child becomes a member of the nanny's family. This means it is neither the nanny becoming a member of Vietnamese family, nor the parents becoming members of the nanny's family. This model is seen in the case of Khanh and her grandma. As the following account makes evident, "becoming part of grandma's kinship" is much more than just using kinship terminology and becoming friends with nanny's friends and relatives. To *be kinned* means to feel included in the kinship, *subject to the common kin trajectory*. The social dimension of kinship creates "continuity over time and gives people a sense of belonging to a 'life' to something bigger than the individual" (Howell, 2003, p.466).

> When we went to Aunt Jana, it was automatic that I said hello to her and went to the room to play with their children. And we went together to the cemetery and I was curious about who is this and that is. And my granny told me "this is great grandmother." And I said "wow, really?" Then I came home and told my mum that in the cemetery there is our great grandmother.

Feeling a shared kin trajectory with grandmas and interpreting their position within this trajectory was quite often articulated in the interviews with children. As the introductory story of Minh at the beginning of this chapter has indicated, unconscious reference to the nanny's genealogy was part of the broader process in which children gave meaning and a sense of the ties in which they lived. Such testimonies reflect the children's understanding of kinship and belonging to a kinned trajectory. Howell argues (2003, p.466) in her research on adoptees that through the process of kinning, children are enrolled in a kinned trajectory that overlaps with that of their adopted parents. Similarly, some Vietnamese children who are looked after by Czech nannies are brought into their nannies' kinned trajectory. However, this trajectory is only one of two trajectories which the children are part of. As the "grandchildren" of Czech "grandmas," and the offspring of their own biological parents and grandparents, these Vietnamese children are part of two kinned trajectories—each based on different and distinct grounds, emotions, and senses of belonging (see Chapter 6).

5.2.1.2 Ms. Orlová: "With them I feel more like a grandma"

In July 2011 I met Ms. Orlová, a 70-year-old widow living in a village with two dogs and a cat. Ms. Orlová warmly welcomed me in her house where she has been living "since forever," and where she brought up two sons of her own. One of them lives not far from her in the same village, and hence she is in a regular contact both with him and her grandchildren. We arranged the appointment on the phone, at which time Ms. Orlová mentioned that her granddaughter would be there when I arrived. We sat in the kitchen and Ms. Orlová offered me her homemade cake. I immediately asked where her granddaughter was. "She is playing in the living room," replied Ms. Orlová and, called her to come to see me. A 14-year-old Vietnamese girl (called Diu) entered the kitchen, sat next to me and they both started describing what they had done yesterday and what their plan for tomorrow was. It as mid-summer and Diu was spending her holiday at grandma's. When she was younger, however, it was not only the holidays that she spent with her nanny; Diu had also been a live-in child for a couple of years with her nanny. Like almost all the nannies in my sample, Ms. Orlová stressed during the interview that she treated Diu "like her own grandchildren," and explained the main difference between grandmothering her son's children and grandmothering Diu:

> I would say that I feel more like a grandma with her because I could not be with my own grand-children when they were small (…) I was not here the whole day, I was working in the city and they were here. When I came home from work, I went to them, of course, but I was not in daylong touch.

Intensive contact between nanny and child leads to a transformation of the concept of grandmotherhood on the part of the nannies who have already experienced grandmothering with their children's children. Ms. Orlová's account is very similar to what Khanh described when reflecting on the differences between her Czech and Vietnamese grandmas. What exactly does it mean to feel "more like a grandma," and where does this feeling come from? There are three key factors in developing feelings of grandmotherhood toward a child: 1) the amount of time spent with the child; 2) the age of the child when care-giving starts; and 3) the degree of decisionmaking power the grandmother has regarding the child's care.

Ms. Orlová feels more like a grandma with her Vietnamese grand-children because she spends more time with them than with her biological grandchildren. While for her Czech grandchildren Ms. Orlová is only what she calls a "Sunday grandma," for her Vietnamese grandchildren she is a "full-time grandma." As Ms. Orlová puts it: "In the evening they (the Czech children) went home because they had their parents," she said, while the Vietnamese children stayed in the evening, because their home was her home. While such intense grandmothering diminishes over time as children grow up and require less time being cared for, Czech grandmothers like Ms. Orlová insist that grandmothering their Vietnamese grandchildren is a lifelong activity, and that their mutual ties are permanent due to the common experiences and memories between them.

Ms. Orlová also feels more like a grandma with her Vietnamese grand-children because she began looking after them when they were very little. She recalls the intensity of contact with a small child who is absolutely dependent on her. She had not experienced such dependence since raising her own children (and as stated above, never with grandchildren), Diu was 12 months old when she became live-in child. Some nannies reported feeling an enormous responsibility when agreeing to look after such small children; however, as discussed in Chapter 5, their own mothering experiences provided them with the skills and knowledge needed to take care of new born babies.

Third and finally, Ms. Orlová feels more like grandma with her Vietnamese grand-children because she is their primary care-giver. Like Khanh's grandma, Ms. Orlová is a fulltime grandmother, and is responsible for the children every day, all day long. "It was everything—doctors, insurance, I knew more about them than their parents," says Ms. Orlová, recalling the period when the children lived with her, and their parents came to see them only on Saturdays for two or three hours. The strong ties between her and her Vietnamese granddaughter and grandson continue, even though contact is now limited to occasional visits, Christmas, and vacations. During vacation time, Ms. Orlová again becomes a full-time grandmother, with the parents coming to visit only a few times during the two month vacation period. After each of the times spent together, saying goodbye is very emotional. Dui still cries when she leaves her grandma, and Ms. Orlová admits that during vacation she gets used to having the child with her, and has difficulty readjusting to being with without her once vacation ends.

5.2.2 Package Two: Ritual Family Activities

"Ritual family activities" is the second umbrella category under which I put the activities which had special meanings for interviewees and for their family life. Generally there are two kinds of meanings that lead me to call these activities "ritual." First, there are what I call "liminal (transitional) moments" in the life of a cared-for child in which the nanny participates. These include such events as enrolment in kindergarten/primary school or the first day at school. For instance, Khanh and Bui recalled going to their first day at school with mother, father and nanny. Khanh recounted how nice it was to be with both her parents and her grandma on such an important day. Bui added that her parents wanted her "aunt" (the nanny) to go with them, not only because they were afraid that without her they would not understand the teacher, but because for the parents her presence confirmed her importance in the family and in Bui's life. Such liminal activities also work in the opposite direction, in that the children and their parents are part of the liminal moments in the nannies' lives. Trai recalled his Czech grandfather's funeral, where he, his sister, and parents were considered members of the nanny's family, to whom others expressed their condolences.

Then there are "family building" activities which strengthen the sense of familial belonging and emotional ties. These include important days of the year, such as Christmas and birthdays, or school performances. Nannies are commonly invited to celebrations within the Vietnamese community (the lunar New Year, marriages, birthday celebrations, etc.) and their attendance is very important to the children and their families. Bui told me that it was common for school performances to be attended by three people—the mother, the father and the nanny. She also remembers that while the parents alternated in the audience (one year the father would come, the next year the mother), her nanny was *always* there.

The presence of the nanny at significant events is important for cared-for Vietnamese children, as the following account by 16-year-old Mia, makes clear. Mia was the youngest of my interviewees when we in 2010 at a café in the center of the town where she lives. Her parents have a shop just a few meters from the place where we were sitting and drinking coffee. Mia spoke kindly about her grandmother, who had been looking after her and her younger sister and brother since Mia was four months old. Before she became her nanny, Ms. Májová (about 50 years old) was unemployed. Mia's parents persuaded her to take care of Mai, and later, to take care of her sister and brother. According to Mai, at first Ms.

Májová did not want to look after the brother because "she felt old." However, "they [her Czech grandma and grandpa] realized that we would find someone else and they would lose us all," and so she agreed to bring up all three siblings. The fact that all three children have had the same Czech grandmother has been an important factor in creating a sense of belonging to a single kinship unit (contrary to the quite common experience of fragmentation in cases where each child in the family has a different nanny).

I conducted my interview with Mia in the middle of vacation, and when I asked her whether she was still in touch with her grandma, she replied "of course" and that she came to see her regularly, once or twice a week. At the time of the interview, Ms. Májová was no longer working as a nanny, as Mia was now able to take care of her 10-year-old sister and 7-year-old brother. The children continue to celebrate birthdays with their former nanny, as well as Christmas—a holiday that according to Mia is inconceivable without her "grandmother."

> Mia: We are always with them on Christmas and have carp and potato salad [a typical Czech Christmas meal].
>
> Adéla: So right on Christmas Eve?
>
> Mia: Yes.
>
> Adéla: So there are many of you there …
>
> Mia: Grandmother, our family, that's five people, and then her daughter with her husband and two kids. Ten people together. Besides they take the dogs …
>
> Adéla: It must be awesome, with a big tree. And it's been this way since childhood?
>
> Mia: Since childhood, we spent Christmas there with my granny. To be honest, I cannot imagine the Christmas atmosphere at home because in Vietnam Christmas is not celebrated much, so …

Mia's account reveals both the importance of celebrating Christmas together (inseparability of particular events from the presence of the grandmother), as well as the performative aspect of this event. The fact that Christmas is celebrated with nanny and *her family* makes Mia and her own family part of the nanny's family.

There was another reason why both children and nannies emphasized the role of Christmas and birthday parties in their lives and in their relationship: gift-giving. For my interviewees, gift-giving is a two-way, reciprocal act that symbolizes the mutuality, reciprocity, and authenticity of the relationship between nanny and child. Gift-giving is evoked as support for statements like "the nanny does not do it for money" or "you cannot do it for money," and taken as proof that nanny and child are bound not by economic transactions (that of employer-employee), but by pure and sincere kinship ties.

5.2.3 Package Three: Exclusive Czech Grandma Activities

The third and final set of activities are those I call "exclusive Czech grandma activities." These refer to activities that children said they could do *only* with their Czech grandmothers. Contrary to the first group of activities (parents-responsibility substitute activities),—which were done by the nanny *instead of by the* parents—or to the second group of activities (ritual family activities), which were performed *with* parents, children referred to a third group of activities that could only be performed with grandma, and *not* with parents. The "exclusive" nature of this third set of activities stemmed from the nanny's ethnic background (as a Czech) and from the fact that these activities could not be done with their biological grandparents because of the physical distance from Vietnam. The case of Yen (described below) illustrates this point well, as well as how the children in my sample understand kinship ties between themselves and their grandmothers in the Czech Republic and in Vietnam. Similarly, some nannies were able to experience with their Vietnamese grandchildren what they could not experience with their biological grandchildren—what I call intensive "grandmothering." The example of Ms. Havranová illuminates such subjectivation of nanny to grandmother.

5.2.3.1 Yen: "you can say you have a grandma"

Yen was 20 years old when we met. She and her younger brother were born in the Czech Republic and had had a Czech grandmother since their childhood. Though her contact with her grandmother had become less intense as she was attending university in another city, Yen always found time to visit her grandmother and have tea with her. When recalling her childhood and the role of the Czech nanny in her life, Yen reported:

> You know Czech things like the picking mushrooms, working in the garden, Czech fairy tales. But the most important thing I felt those days was that I just had a grandma. When kids say "I'm going to grandma's," so I also had such a grandma. You know sometimes it is hard to stay here only with mum and you have no other support. That is what I felt when I was small. Now I rely on myself, but before I just felt that with grandma, I had some kind of certainty and support.

Yen's account makes apparent what was already outlined above—that there are some activities which children consider reserved exclusively for their Czech grandmothers. One such activity is spending vacations at the grandmother's home. This activity acquires a special status in child interviewee accounts. In Yen's account this is the most evident when she talks about working in the grandmother's garden and picking mushrooms. "In my childhood I could hoe the vegetables and when I found an earthworm, I started screaming, and grandma came and threw it away." Yen's vacations, like those of other interviewees, epitomized the close connection between child and grandmother, and the grandmother becomes the symbol of childhood. Imbued with special meaning, vacation at grandmas' often represents for child and nanny, alike, the essence of "grandchildhood" and "grandmotherhood."

"Grandma exclusive" activities are understood by children as those activities they can experience only with the *Czech* grandmother. As Yen argues, they are those "Czech things" that could not be experienced with her mother because her mother was not familiar with them, but that are somehow important for living in Czech society. Picking mushrooms was repeated in many interviews as an example of what children perceived as a typical Czech activity that they enjoyed doing with their grandmas. In this regard, the grandma provides children with what we could call a "door to majority" (paraphrasing Rollins' "window to exotica; Rollins, 1985; Souralová, 2014b). The nanny as a mediator of "Czech culture" offers and teaches children Czech habits and traditions (most often mentioned were Advent, Easter, but also events like pig-slaughtering). The children in my sample place tremendous emphasis on the role of the nanny in acquiring direct and personal contact with the Czech environment, which they consider as one of the most important aspects of their childhood. Many children concluded that while they *knew a great deal* about Czech culture and traditions from school and friends, it was through their nannies that they were able to *live* these traditions and experience them as *authentic*. Thanks to their grandmothers, these children "learned to adapt" (as Bui put it) to Czech society.

"But the most important thing I felt those days was that I had a grandma," stated Yen, stressing the significant aspect of her relationship with her nanny. Similarly, Minh (whose story was introduced at the beginning of this chapter) emphasized the role of his grandmother, Ms. Kosová, with the following words: "It is, you know, that you just can say 'I have a grandma,' just the word." While Yen's words refer to the need to share geographical closeness with one's grandmother (you can "go" to your grandmother), Minh's comments highlights the symbolic *need* to have a grandmother. A need which in theory could be fulfilled—but is not—by the biological grandmother in Vietnam. The question then is why is the need for "having a grandma" not satisfied by simply having Vietnamese grandmothers in Vietnam? Both Yen and Minh have their biological grandmothers in Vietnam. Yet their need to have and to be able to go to a grandma can only be accomplished with a Czech grandmother. This fact brings to the fore an essential element in the grandchild-Czech grandmother relationship: the geographical and symbolic displacement of children from their Vietnamese grandmothers.

Yen's account reveals the consequences of *physical displacement*—the spatial distance between her and her grandmothers in Vietnam. The saying "going to grandma's" is impossible to connect to the Vietnamese grandmother, as she is 8,000 km away, and going to her requires overcoming spatial, financial, and cultural (language) barriers. Even though Yen is part of the transnational social field via relatively regular phone calls, her need for spatial closeness and a "here-and-now grandchildhood" is accomplished only with her Czech grandmother, who comes to substitute the Vietnamese grandmother in the role of care-giver and grandmother.

Minh's statement that "you can say that you have a grandma" takes us even further into the concept of kinship. For Minh and other interviewees, it is not only the spatial barrier that leads them to acknowledge the role of the Czech grandmother. It is above all the fact that the children's biological grandmothers do not figure in the children's mental maps as true grandmothers. Or more precisely, Vietnamese grandmothers are overshadowed by Czech grandmothers. *Symbolic displacement* of the Vietnamese grandmothers is palpable throughout my sample, particularly when it comes to the definitions and associations children have about "the grandmother." When I asked Hue, a 22-year-old woman born in the Czech Republic, how she would define "who is grandmother," she replied:

> Hue: Well, I would say, because I am trained at university to think rationally, then I would say that it is the mother's mother. But if I had to elaborate it more … wow, I do not know, when I think about it, I feel like I direct it to my Czech grandma. So the grandmother is someone who takes care of you and you have some emotional ties so that it is not just anybody who does her job and is paid for it. It must be based on the relationship. But now I talk about my Czech grandma. Well, with the Vietnamese grandma it is the same but it is not paid (laughs).
>
> Adéla: So the main difference between the Czech and Vietnamese grandmother is that one is paid and other is not?
>
> Hue: Well, rather no. I had no association with my Vietnamese grandma; the only thing which came in my mind was connected to my Czech grandma and then I started thinking what to say on behalf of the Vietnamese one.

In Hue's account, the symbolic displacement of the Vietnamese grandmothers is manifest in the absence of mental associations with them. There is nothing to say about these grandmothers—the only associations are connected to genealogy, namely that they are their parents' mothers. However, symbolic displacement by no means implies the total erasing of Vietnamese grandparents. As Chapter 6 will show, the figure of the Vietnamese grandmother plays an essential role in the way children imagine belonging to a kinship genealogy and to a national homeland. Reference to the parents' mothers was very present in the interviews; children called them their "real," "birth," or "blood" grandmothers. The symbolic power of biogenetic conceptions of kinship is of huge importance to children whose "real" grandmothers cannot spend time with them. These children feel compelled to defend the reality of their ties with Czech nannies, both to themselves and to other people—as Khanh says:

> I was six or seven years old, and when I went somewhere, I went there with my granny. And I told everyone around that she is my granny. The children told me she could not be my granny because we are not alike. Then I was crying a lot and I kept on saying that she was my granny. My parents had to explain to me that she is not my granny and that she only looks after me and that my grannies were in Vietnam. And those days I was split because I told them "the grannies in Vietnam are not my grannies because they never looked after me, they have never been with me and they have never spent time with me. They even do not know what I like!

Children's reflections illuminate the tensions in understanding family and kinship ties, and reveal two conceptions of kinship definition. This excerpt suggests that the distinction between the Czech and Vietnamese grandmother is based on four essential and intertwined dualities which we can summarize in the following way:

Immediate care for and care about versus care about at distance
Khanh's account shows that there is an enormous difference between the Czech grandmother—who *cares for* her (looks after her and "goes everywhere" with her) and *cares about her* (knows what Khanh likes)—and the Vietnamese grandmothers, who have *never* cared for her, and whose ability to care about her is limited by physical distance. Khanh's statement that "The grannies in Vietnam are not my grannies because they have never looked after me," reflects the element of "care" as the main structuring factor in her kinship relationship with her Czech grandmother. In other words, the children's understanding of kinship starts with the issue of caring, according to which Vietnamese and Czech grandmothers are measured and compared. While children recognized that their grandmothers in Vietnam surely loved them and cared about them (were interested in their lives and supported their success, etc.), children felt more bonded to their Czech grandmas, who cared for them on an everyday basis.

Performance for versus existence of the relationship
The emphasis on care-giving in the definition of kinship parallels the age-old discussion of whether blood is thicker than water. Previously I said that active time with the Czech grandmother was contrasted with the lack of time—especially of quality time—spent with parents. A similar contrast is made when comparing Czech and Vietnamese grandmothers, such as when Khanh says "Vietnamese grannies are not my grannies." However, in other places in the interview she is less categorical in her declarations, and (like other children) is able to distinguish between kinship through performance and kinship through existence. Khanh's reckoning indicates that the difference in feelings is based on the dichotomy of "real" versus "created through caring": "Above all, I have absolutely different feelings for my grandma who was caring for me and for my real grandmas. Definitely. I know that they are my family but I do not have such deep feelings for them as I have for this granny who took care of me." In Khanh's view, "real"

means based on blood, genes, and genealogy, which has the symbolic power to tell the story of one's roots. "Somewhere deep inside I know I have my Vietnamese grandmothers," is a common statement of child interviewees, and reflects the symbolism of blood relations in kinship ties. These blood relations do not transcend spatial distance nor provide children with daily face-to-face grandmothering—but they are present, deep in the children's heart, and may be awakened and "lived" anytime. Kinship ties with Czech grandmothers, on the other hand, do not exist a priori, but are the result of daily practices. They are not awakened, but rather created and recreated through the process of kinning.

Absence of shared history versus absence of shared memory

Vietnamese grandmothers figure in the children's accounts as their parents' parents. Reference to genealogy is the one element in the grandmother-grandchild relationship that the Czech grandmother cannot provide. So while children feel they belong to the kinned trajectory of their Czech grandmas (as discussed in case of Khanh), these feelings contrast with feelings of belonging to a genealogy and shared kinned history, which can only be provided by their biological grandmothers. In other words, while the Czech grandmothers are the reservoir of memories and connections to their social networks, Vietnamese grandmothers connect children with their kinship network—aunts, uncles, cousins, etc.—whose strength lies in the imagination of common ancestors and roots (as Chapter 6 will further elaborate). "Being a Nguyen" (like the generations before) gives children *continuity over time* and hence a source of safety and sense of belonging.

Direct relationship versus parents-mediated relationship

The final difference in the two conceptions of kinship is based on the degree of personal experience of being kinned. The fact that the Vietnamese grandmothers are described through genealogy (as noted above) also indicates that children define their relations with them through their relations with parents. Simply put, their ties are always mediated by a third actor—the parent; the relationship with Vietnamese grandmothers is based on the logic *child → parents → grandparents*. On the other hand, the ties with Czech grandmothers are always created directly between the child and the nanny. The parents are usually not part of this kinning process, and hence not part of the kinship relations between the child and the Czech grandmother. The ties with Czech grandmothers instead follow the equation *child ↔ grandparents*.

For Yen's mother, Yen's Czech grandmother is not like a second mother; Yen described her mother and Czech grandmother's relationship as friendly and warm, but limited by language competencies. When I asked Yen whether her mother would go to her grandmother for help when she had any problems, she replied "no, she would rather go to the Vietnamese." When I asked her where she—Yen—would go if any problems emerged, she replied to her grandma. This was already apparent in her account above, where she said that "sometimes it is hard to stay when you are here only with mum and you have no other support." This aspect of grandma-grandchild ties will be important in Chapter 6.

5.2.3.2 Ms. Havranová: "I can be grandma with him"

In this chapter I discussed the fact that the motivation for many women in my sample to become nannies after retiring was because the work afforded them inter-generational bonding. Some women wanted to experience more intensive grandmothering than they were able to have with their children's children; others longed to experience grandmothering before having any grandchildren of their own. One nanny in my sample, Ms. Havranová, had not had any grandchildren of her own and she could not even have any in the future. When she retired, her only son became seriously ill and needed fulltime daycare, which she and professional nurses provided. Around that time, a Vietnamese family contacted Ms. Havranová, asking whether she could take care of a six-month-old boy named Chien. At the beginning it was quite difficult for her to balance her time between her son and Chien. Within a short time, however, the little boy became her greatest balm, and helped her and her husband to deal with their emotionally difficult family situation. Ms. Havranová recalled this situation by saying:

> It was very hard for us because our son was bedridden. And my husband had to start visiting the psychiatrist. And he once told me 'you know, when the little boy put his arms around me and hugs me, that is better than a thousand pills.' (…) And then our son passed away two years ago so now we have Chien because we do not have our own grand-children. So we have him like our own and we spoil him very much.

The strong emotional ties between Ms. Havranová, her husband and Chien, developed when the couple were dealing with the loss of their only son. Looking back, Ms. Havranová emphasizes the importance of the little boy's presence in their life. Chien gave their life new meaning, and they bestowed on the boy all the love that they would have invested in their own son.

When Chien started attending kindergarten, the paid care-giving was terminated. Soon afterwards, however, Ms. Havranová asked Chien's parents if she and her husband could still see Chien *from time to time*, as she had grown used to the boy's presence and wanted to stay in touch with him. The parents agreed, and Ms. Havranová and her husband began picking him up from kindergarten. Soon, "from time to time" became "everyday," and Chien quickly became Ms. Havranová's "darling," (to use her words). Chien also became Ms. Havranová's greatest pride, as she put all her energy into her relationship with him. When Chien was in fifth grade, he took part in the regional round of SCIO testing in Mathematics and Czech. He placed 17th in Mathematics and first in Czech. Afterwards he said, "It's because I have you, granny." Ms. Havranová described with happiness that she—a former Czech language teacher—had been able to help *her* boy succeed in her beloved discipline.

Ms. Havranová's relationship with Chien was now even stronger, and greatly affected her life trajectory. When her own son finally passed away, she and her husband were forced to find a new housing arrangement, as their personal finances did not allow them to stay in the same apartment. The couple found an apartment quite far from the city where they had lived. Ms. Havranová described how Chien "had a fit," started crying, and begged them not to leave him. Chien's father mobilized his social networks and found a new family for his son's grandmother. When Chien later found out that his grandmother would stay in the city, he was very happy. Later, however, he learned that that his grandmother would be living with some girls, and he began crying again, convinced that she had exchanged him for other children. They had to explain to him that he would always be their only grandson, and that they would never stop loving him. Though Ms. Havranová is growing older, and would at times prefer to have more time to herself (to be able to "take a bath and not only a quick shower in the evening"), she still makes her decisions around what she perceives as best for Chien, as the following words suggest: "I am tired and I still struggle with myself whether I should move to the village or not. But I was born here, I have my heart here. And above all I have Chien here, so maybe later when he is more independent."

This account in particular shows that the entire biography of Ms. Havranová is shaped by her care-giving of the boy. It is an absolute transformation of her biography to grandmothering, or more accurately said, her *subjectivation* to the role of grandmother (on subjectivation and kinship see Faubion, 2001). Of all the roles in her repertoire (wife, friend, sister), it is the role of grandmother that is performed at the expense of other roles. In fact, only the role of wife is perfectly compatible with the role of grandmother, as Ms. Havranová's husband has also become Chien's grandfather and the performance of other roles is limited. This subjectivation occurs, as I already mentioned above, only between children and nannies (and their partners/families). The parents are excluded. The case of Ms. Havranová also illuminates the vast discrepancy in intimacy and depth between the nanny's relationship with the child, and her relationship with the child's parents. This discrepancy is especially apparent in the divergent manner in which Ms. Havranová refers to the parents and to the child: When speaking about Chien's father she refers to "Mr. Engineer and his family," while when speaking about the boy, she refers to "our Chien." When asked about her relationship to the father and boy, Ms. Havranová responded: We are on formal terms with each other (referring to her relationship with the father), but the boy is ours."

* * *

Intensive daily care-giving lays the groundwork for the creation of kinship relations between nannies (grandmothers) and children (grandchildren). Kinning is a long-term process which contains various activities and leads to the creation of permanent ties based on mutuality, reciprocity, and emotion between grandchild and grandmother. It is too soon to know whether these relationships based on care will also operate in the opposite direction, with the Vietnamese grandchildren providing care to their Czech grandmothers when the latter begin to need it. However, what is clear is that children—and to a lesser extent their nannies—negotiate two sets of kinship conceptions—biogenetic and performative. While for Czech nannies such negotiations are usually straightforward and simple—the nannies just say "I treat them like my own"—for children the balancing between two concepts of kinship ties is part of broader answer to the essential question of "where do I belong?" and "who am I?."

Chapter 6
"Europe is My Brain, Asia is My Heart": GrandMotherland and Kinning as Home-Bonding

"Homeland is where my family lives."

Kim, an 18-year-old Vietnamese girl

My name is Yen and I am one of many second generation Vietnamese children living in the Czech Republic. I am 19 years old now and I have just started my university studies. My parents came to the Czechoslovakia in the late 1980s, where they met and later married. Like other Vietnamese immigrants they started their business, and since they did not have enough time for me and my younger brother, they found a nanny for us. Sometimes it is hard for us in the Czech Republic. For my mum it is hard because she spends her life earning money. She has no leisure time, only working, working, working. And for me it is hard because I feel like a stranger. We do not have family here, and my friends cannot understand me fully.

My mum wants to return to Vietnam later when we—me and my brother—are adults and have our own families. We have only been to Vietnam once in my whole life. Neither us nor our mum has had the opportunity to go there more often because it is quite expensive. I remember our visit to Vietnam as though it were yesterday. Four years ago we went there to meet our relatives. I felt like a stranger there, which was weird because I expected to feel at home there. But it was not so. Again—as in the Czech Republic—I felt like a foreigner and people recognized at first sight that I was from Europe. I did not have to open my mouth to say anything; they just looked at me and saw it. I do not understand how. But what was the biggest experience for me was to see how my mum changed when we were in Vietnam. I can say that it was the first time I saw my mum happy. She was so happy to be there! But it lasted only a couple of days and then we returned to the Czech Republic and she started working again.

I do not have these ties to Vietnam, as my mum does. I do not even like the Vietnamese community living in the Czech Republic. Since I was growing up with my Czech grandma and surrounded by Czech peers, I was slowly losing my knowledge of the Vietnamese language. And it is quite hard to speak with Vietnamese people here because they usually judge you. And when you speak Vietnamese with a Czech accent, they look down on you. When I was younger, my Czech grandma was a big support for me. Not only because she initiated me into Czech society—we did those typical Czech things together like picking mushrooms and so on—but because she was always there for me. I just felt a kind of certainty with her and I knew I could turn to her if I had any problem. When I was a child, it was important to know that there was another person besides my mum in whom I could trust and confide. Now I am an adult, so I am independent and can solve all my problems by myself.

As I said, my friends rarely understand me. I mean my Czech friends—how could they when they do not have the experience of being second generation immigrant? If I had Vietnamese friends, they would not understand me either. Only one friend is on the same wavelength as I am—and it is because she is a second generation Vietnamese too. We are banana kids: Inside we are Czech because we have lived here all our lives, but outside we are Vietnamese, and we cannot do anything about it. And even if we did not care, people would remind us that we are not Czechs. Actually, I am not sure whether I am both Czech and Vietnamese, or neither Czech nor Vietnamese. Are my homelands both the Czech Republic and Vietnam, or neither the Czech Republic nor Vietnam?

* * *

The question of belonging is one of the most important issues that my child interviewees confront. When I asked them how they would define their homeland, they very often referred to a family or kinship network—stating that "homeland is where my family is." As the previous chapter showed, the notion of family is quite ambiguous for children of Vietnamese parents who are brought up by Czech nannies—and so is the question of belonging. The story of Yen depicts the crucial issues which emerge when it comes to the question of "who I am" and "where do I belong." These issues, which will be elaborated in this chapter and include the role of the Czech grandmother in feelings of belonging, and the role of parents and Vietnamese grandparents as well as Vietnam itself in longing to belong.

Several research studies have focused on the practice of belonging, and on how second generation immigrants imagine the homeland (Espiritu, 2003; Levitt and Walters, 2002, and so on). In this chapter I focus on one particular aspect of belonging: the significance of kinship in giving children "a sense of belonging to something bigger than the individual" (Howell, 2003, p.466). I focus on how the strength of emotional attachment to kin and ideas about belonging to the national homeland are mediated and transmitted through kinship ties. Both kinds of stories—the story of kinning and the story of belonging—provoke deep emotions when being told. This is because they are stories not only about emotional attachment, but also about identification, the narration of self, and about the position of self in social relationships and the world.

I have put the word "GrandMotherland" in the title of this chapter to prefigure my argument and explore how narratives of kinship and belonging are similar with respect to language, metaphor, and explanation. Having dealt earlier with the process of kinning, in this chapter I look at the consequences of the ambivalent kinship concepts for belonging, imagining, and feeling at home. In section 6.1, I present three case studies in order to show the intra-action of narratives of kinship and of belonging. These case studies are further summarized in section 6.2, where I focus specifically on the symbolism of kinship and belonging, and on intergenerational perspectives of belonging.

6.1 Belonging in/through Kinship: Three Case Studies

In this section, I profile three second generation individuals whom I selected because they present three distinct patterns in the imagination of homeland. In all three cases, individuals express strong, spontaneous, emotional statements about kinship, forming the centre of their sense of belonging. I selected these particular individuals in order to portray the diverse and often contradictory manner in which these Vietnamese children speak about kinship and homeland. Differences in their imagination of homeland is conditioned by several critical factors: 1) The place of birth and/or age of the child when arriving in the Czech Republic; 2) the child's current age; and 3) the child's engagement in the maintenance of transnational ties; i.e. their transnational kinship ties negotiations.

As Peggy Levitt (2002, p.139) argues, "transnational activities do not remain constant across the life cycle. Instead, they ebb and flow at different stages, varying with the demands of work, school, and family." In this section I look at three children—Hanh, Tuyet, and Trai—whose home-bonds were shaped under very different conditions, and were told at different life stages. Hanh was 18 years old when I interviewed her. She exhibits the pattern of the Vietnamese child born in the Czech Republic, for whom Vietnam figures as the parents' place of birth. Tuyet was 21 years old when I interviewed her, and had come to the Czech Republic from Vietnam at the age of three. For Tuyet, Vietnam figures not only as the birthplace of her parents but also as *her* birthplace (though she has no actual memory of living there). Trai, for his part, was 25 years old at the time of our interview, and had come to the Czech Republic at the age of seven. Having spent more years in Vietnam than Tuyet and Hanh, Trai considered Vietnam not only his and his parents' place of birth, but also as a place in his personal history.

6.1.1 Hanh: Kinship and Belonging in Motion

"Something about me? That I am frustrated all the time, indeed." So began my two hour talk with Hanh, an 18-year-old-girl, born in the Czech Republic. Later in her account she used the word "frustration" once again to explain what leads her to think about herself in these terms. "The biggest problem I have with myself is the frustration of not knowing where I belong, to what family I belong." Hanh presented herself explicitly as a "split personality." This split was apparent in the ambivalence of her account as well as in the vocabulary she used. In the quotation above, Hanh says that she has a "problem with herself," instead of saying "My problem is." While this interview was exceptional—both in terms of its content and emotionality—, it addressed an issue that was present in all my interviews with child interviewees: the ambiguity of belonging through kinship ties, particularly when these ties are unclear and complex.

Early on in the interview Hanh said, "I have no home." Later she stated, "I feel more at home in the Czech Republic than in Vietnam, but not fully at home." These statements reflected the tenor of the entire interview. When I asked Hanh what came into her mind when she said the word "home," she replied (after a short hesitation) "family." When I asked what Vietnam meant to her, her description flew from the parents (as her point of reference) to kinship ties, oscillating between those with her relatives in Vietnam and those with her Czech grandmother in the Czech Republic:

> Hanh: My parents' place of birth. It is simply what my parents took from me because I was born here. I just feel so sorry because my mum has a huge family—she had seven siblings. I feel sorry for the children in Vietnam that they did not have the chance to enjoy as much as I could, they had more obligations than me, their lives were not easy but they had what I have never had. They came home and they had family. They came to grandma and they had their own grandma, nothing simulated or artificial. And they had their own background. (…)
>
> Adéla: You said simulated, how did you mean that?
>
> Hanh: I meant that they had their birth grandma who knows all the members of the family, and all your cousins and ancestors, and it is the real family. I take my Czech grandma more as a grandmother than my Vietnamese grandmothers, right? Than the real ones. And I can never tell them. And of course I know that they cannot love me as much as they love the other granddaughters of theirs. They have had the opportunity to get to know them. I know that when some of my friends were born their grandparents were already not around. But the worst thing is that mine are here and I have no way of getting to know them.

This quotation reveals several important issues in Hanh's imagination about her homeland and its connection to kinship. When Hanh says that "Vietnam is my parents' birthplace," and that "Vietnam is the home that was taken from me," she is expressing what she understands to be a homeland and "birth" or "real" kinship ties. This contrasts with her understanding of her home and family life in the Czech Republic, which she considers "artificial" and "simulated," yet in many respects more "real" than her family in Vietnam. To better understand these two important issues, I will focus here on *emic understandings of kinship and belonging as the negotiation between "artificial" and "real,"* and the *moment of motion in her imagination of homeland.*

First is *the imagination of what is home, based on the tension between "artificial" and "birth."* This is the leitmotif of Hanh's self-perception as a frustrated person that has "no home." Hanh did not feel split and uprooted all her life. "I always felt like a little Czech," recalled Hanh, whose Czech grandmother began caring for her when she was only 18 months old. "When I started kindergarten, I had my Czech grandma, Czech friends, and I felt that I was living a normal life. When someone asked me where I was from, I simply replied that that I was Czech. I never said I was Vietnamese—I was simply Czech, I was living here and would be living here forever." Hanh's feeling of belonging to the Czech Republic were unproblematic and natural. The role of her Czech grandmother in this period was crucial. "I knew I had my (Vietnamese) grandmother, but my only grandma was her (Czech nanny), just her," emphasized Hanh. In her account, Hanh describes the importance of her Czech grandma in her childhood in the following manner:

> I can say that she gave me a home then. Now she cannot give it to me anymore because I think differently about things. But before she was simply my home. Because of her I did not want to leave the Czech Republic. You know, not because of my friends or the teachers at school that I liked, but because of my granny. Because my granny was here for me … she was home for me.

It was quite common for the children I interviewed to link grandmother and home; however, "home" in these cases meant "family," family life, and the background which provided children with a feeling of security. Only in some cases was the notion of family directly connected to the country. In the case of Hanh, however, "home" meant "homeland." "Because of her (Czech grandmother) I did not want to leave the Czech Republic," says Hanh, making it clear that her kinship ties with her Czech grandmother are grounds for establishing ties with the country. Similar to what Diane Wolf (2002) describes as "emotional transnationalism," here we can see what I call "emotional localism," which provides Hanh with local and intergenerational points of reference based on emotional attachments and intergenerational ties developed and situated in the Czech Republic. These reference points are ties that bind, that act as a source of membership, and that provide reasons for staying or returning to a particular place or country.

In Hanh's account, "emotional localism" thwarts the existence of emotional transnationalism at a particular stage of childhood.

> When I was seven years old, we went for the second time in my life to Vietnam. I came to my [Czech] grandma and I was so happy that I would see my real grandparents and I told her "Granny, I am going to see my grandmas and grandpas!" And she was crying so much. I remember how much she was crying because she was afraid I was going to realize that I was not her granddaughter. We were calling her from Vietnam and calming her because she could not stop crying. And when I was in Vietnam, we went to my grandmother on mother's side. When I saw her, she was not at all as beautiful as my Czech grandma, she was different. In Vietnam they were chewing betel and it makes your teeth red. And when I saw her, Jesus, what kind of monster she was, she was not my grandma! She wanted to cuddle me but I simply said that she was not my

> grandmother. I counted on my grandma going with us to Vietnam, and when I saw I had no place there, I cried, and I missed her so much.

The depth of emotional feeling between Hanh and her Czech grandmother is clearly expressed in this account, and contrasts with later statements by Hanh that her ties to the Czech grandmother are "simulated" or "artificial." While Hanh initially presents her Czech grandmother as someone providing help, understanding, and a sense of place, later on Hanh appears to see her as less important and valuable. Why? What causes such a profound change in Hanh's perception of her Czech grandma, and of her grandmother's place in her life?

I argue (and the first excerpt from interview with Hanh indicates this) that it is because the bonds between Hanh and her Czech grandmother—no matter how emotionally strong—cannot provide Hanh what kinship ties with her Vietnamese grandmother are able to provide. To understand this, we must first examine the change in Hanh's perception of her place within Czech society. "And as I grew older, I started noticing that people look at me differently. They do not even have to say anything, but you can recognize it in the way they look at you," recounts Hanh, in her recollections of childhood. Hanh's observations reflect the changeability of her imagination of homeland, as well as the maintenance of transnational ties during the course of her life (see Levitt, 2002). Hanh's words make evident the profound changes in her imagination of homeland, and the deficiencies of her previous imagination of homeland and kinship ties.

What is the advantage of the belonging-story that the Vietnamese grandmother can tell and the Czech grandmother cannot? In Hanh's description, her Vietnamese grandmother is presented as the trunk of the tree, the base of the kinship: she keeps the family together and is the center from which all other family branches stem. She speaks about a "birth grandma who knows all the members of the family, and all your cousins and ancestors." At the same time—because the Vietnamese grandmother is the trunk of the tree—she is strongly and deeply *rooted* in the soil, in the country of Vietnam. Here the metaphor of family/genealogy takes on solid features and is personified in particular persons—the grandmother—as well as in other relatives. Only through the grandmother and relatives can children access their roots. As I suggest later, children move back and forth between two definitions of kinship: one based on a shared family history, and the other on shared personal memory. This distinction becomes important in how Hanh imagines the homeland. The inadequacy of the personal memory created with the Czech grandmother—who is actually described as a being a more "real" grandmother to Hanh than her birth grandmother—leads Hanh to look for a meta-narrative that tells the story of family ancestors, and that links her to *her* roots. True relatives become those that can provide her clear and stable relationships with other relatives.

Second is *motionality of the imagination of homeland in the accounts* of children who were born in the Czech Republic and visited Vietnam only a few times in their lives. Their narratives of homeland are in motion, as their accounts often follow the time-space logic of origin (coming from), return (coming back to). Between "coming from" and "coming back," there is a liminal/threshold phase in which children—in their effort to define their position in the world—balance between here-there and then-now-after. The *past* is depicted in the children's statements by referring to their *imagination* of their origins. When I asked Mia—a 17-year-old girl—to tell me about herself, she replied, "I am from Vietnam but I was born in the Czech Republic." Hanh answered in a similar fashion, stating that her parents had taken her home from her—meaning that she used to have a home (before she was born), but now does not. Both these examples are manifestations of what Espiritu (1994, p.253, italics added) calls "nostalgic but unacquainted allegiance to an *imagined* past."

The desire for this past is further strengthened by questions about children's origins. As noted above, Hanh was often asked "where are you from." In the early years of her life, this question seemed irrelevant to Hahn. Later on, however, these questions came to shape Hanh's understanding of her position in Czech society. Frank Wu (2002, p.79) describes a similar phenomenon when looking at second-generation Asian Americans:

> "Where are you from?" is a question I like answering. "Where are you *really* from?" is a question I *really* hate answering. (…) For Asian Americans, the questions frequently come paired like that. Among ourselves, we can even joke nervously about how they just about define the Asian-American experience. More than anything else that unites us, everyone with an Asian face who lives in America is afflicted by the perpetual foreigner syndrome. We are figuratively and even literally returned to Asia and ejected from America.

When answering the question "Where are you really from?" Hanh's explanation turns around her parents' past decisions to migrate. The parents transmit two kinds of heritage to Hanh: the heritage of Vietnam (as a possible homeland), and the heritage of migrancy (interpreted as uprootedness and lack of direct contact with family members). These two heritages caused Vietnam to be taken from Hanh when the parents decided to move to the Czech Republic. At the same time, it was not simply the country, but her place in the lineage and clear place in genealogy which were removed from her, even before she had been born. That is why her *present* position and belonging are highly unclear and ambiguous.

The *future* of the homeland is imagined though the narration of return. Hanh says: "I have no place to return to. I cannot return to Czechia, and I cannot return to Vietnam. So where do I return to?" This statement suggests that physical presence (being physically *in* the Czech Republic and physically *with* a Czech grandmother) does not provide Hanh with *enough* to feel a total sense of belonging: Hanh is looking for something stronger and deeper. Her searching is probably nourished by the fact that her parents want to return to Vietnam (as discussed in Chapter 4). In other words, her feeling of belonging is "fed by the parents' nostalgia for the homeland and their dream of returning," as acknowledged by Wessendorf (2007, p.1084), who describes how the sense of belonging and nostalgia for the homeland are transmitted from parents to their second generation immigrant children. It is the nostalgia for the place in the imagined "unproblematic" and "real" kinship trajectory that is not sufficiently fulfilled by the Czech grandmother, as she lacks shared *gene*alogy and connectedness with people who share blood and genes (as other children I interviewed put it).

In summary, in Hanh's account the homeland is imagined as something that *had existed* before being *taken away* from her by parents. Hanh now *misses* this homeland because she feels she has no place where she *can return* to. This perceived loss is emotionally charged, and becomes a source of grief that structures how she imagines her "home," kinship ties, and homeland. It also forces her to look for something that has been lost, instead of appreciating what has been created. Hanh's longing for deep emotional ties with her "real," birth grandmothers, and the realization that such ties are not possible due to physical distance; create feelings of emotional and cultural distance from her Vietnamese kin and homeland.

Hanh, like the other children I interviewed, is not reconciled to her dual identity, nor is her imagination fluid and "settled in mobility" (Morokvasic, 2004). On the contrary, her account (like those of other child interviewees) is pervaded by a desperate desire for solidity, anchoring, and rootedness—both in kinship and in a physical homeland. Hanh is looking for the one steady rock that makes the whole issue of belonging less complicated. Home is personified by the Czech grandmother "who has always been here for me" but who cannot provide a place in kinship genealogy. Therefore Hanh (like other children) later seeks out the Vietnamese grandmother, through whom she imagines she can discover her roots, her relationships with other relatives, and, a complete sense of belonging—both to the kinship trajectory and to the homeland of Vietnam. Hanh's attempts to find her "true roots" are frustrated in the end, as she lacks shared memories, intimate emotions, and the *practice of grandmothering with her Vietnamese grandmother.* In the end, Hanh is left with a feeling of "I do not know where I belong, nor to which family I belong."

6.1.2 Tuyet: Homeland Visits and Kinning the Kinned

Tuyet, a 21-year-old woman, was born in Vietnam. In the 1980s her parents lived in East Germany, and in 1989 decided to return to Vietnam. The boom in the retail business in the Czech Republic led them to immigrate to the Czech Republic, and to settle near the Czech-German border. Tuyet's parents found a nanny for their son and daughter—a retired woman whose children and grandchildren lived far away and did not come to see her very often.

During the interview Tuyet related many memories of her childhood with her Czech nanny- "grandma," who taught her many skills, such as making Christmas candies, or colouring eggs for Easter. A couple of years ago her grandmother passed away, and Tuyet characterized the nature of her ties with her in the following words: "The only grave in the Czech Republic that I visit is in Cheb, where my grandma rests." These words seem to suggest that her former nanny/grandmother serves as Tuyet's connection to the land and culture of the Czech Republic. I would argue that the grave of the Czech grandmother may serve as a connection to the *land*, to the territory of the Czech Republic.

Tuyet's story is noteworthy above all in regard to the significance of her first trip to Vietnam. When this issue came up in the interview, Tuyet replied that it was very difficult for her parents, as they did not earn enough money to buy air tickets for the entire family. This was particularly hard for her parents, whose contact with their family in Vietnam was limited to phone calls. Tuyet described how she communicated with her relatives at that time:

> I was very small when I left Vietnam and I did not remember anything or anybody. So during these ten years [between coming to the Czech Republic and first Vietnam visit] when we used to call to Vietnam, my mum told me 'this is your aunt,' 'this is your uncle' or 'this is your grandma.' When I took the phone, I knew they were my relatives but actually I had no idea who they really are.

Tuyet was part of the transnational social field, maintaining transnational kinship ties with people whom she knew were her relatives, but about whom she knew very little. Her relationship to them (and hence her participation in the transnational social field) was indirect (Lee, 2011), and mediated by the parents, as previously discussed in Chapter 5.

Tuyet's experience is very similar to Hanh's. Both have Czech grandmothers; both refer to their relatives in Vietnam through their parents; and both are growing up as Czechs, with no need to acknowledge the country of their parents' (and Tuyet's) birth. However, the life stories of these two interviewees begin to diverge radically when it comes to the significance of Tuyet's visit to Vietnam. After 10 years living in the Czech Republic, Tuyet's parents said: "Enough, we must go to Vietnam to visit our family." At the age of 13, Tuyet found herself back in the country where she was born, and of which she is a citizen. Eight years after the visit, she described the moment when she met her grandmother in Vietnam after a 10-year separation:

> Well it was very weird because I came there and my mum told me who we were going to see. I did not know these people, they were strangers to me. Then we came to a village where my grandmother, my mother's mother lived. There suddenly a woman took my hand and she was pulling me inside and she was so happy and excited. But I did not know her at all. And she started squeezing my bones, I think she wanted to make sure that I was real or healthy or I don't know. Something like that. So it was interesting. Then after a few minutes or a couple of days maybe I felt the warmth of home, that they were my relatives and my family.

This account reveals the essential role of homeland trips in forming children's understanding of kinship and belonging, and how the idea of the homeland is closely related to kinship ties re-created during visits. I argue here that homeland visits are another kind of family ritual activity (like what was described in Chapter 5) and are part of the kinning process. Howell (2003, p.465–466) emphasizes that "to kin is a universal process, marked in all societies by various rites of passage (…) but it has not generally been recognized as such." A homeland visit is an example of a rite of passage par excellence, and is the main formative force in forging transnational kinship relations. From Tuyet's accounts, it is apparent that her visit to Vietnam transforms the empty word "grandmother" or "aunt" or "uncle" ("I had no idea who they are") into concepts of grandmother, aunt or uncle that evoke meanings, memories, and relationships grounded in personal experience (as opposed to mediated through parents). There is a shift from "a woman I did not know at all" to the "warmth of home," which characterizes the kinning process that occurred during Tuyet's first visit to Vietnam after 10 years of living in the Czech Republic.

King, Christou, and Teerling (2010, p.3) suggest understanding the "homeland visit as a performative act of belonging." Besides the performative act of kinning that occurs during the Vietnam visits, the establishment of emotional ties to the country where relatives live also plays an essential role in creating a sense of belonging. In many accounts the Vietnam visit is interpreted as the *awakening* of latent ties, which are rediscovered during the visit to Vietnam. The encounter with the parents' and grandparents' homeland is experienced very differently by Hanh and Tuyet. While Hanh missed her Czech grandmother and the background she provides her, Tuyet described the spontaneous awareness of kinship ties, which create the "warmth of home." For many of my interviewees, the Vietnam visit marked the turning point in their understanding of their ethnic identity.

The examination of child interviewees' recollections and reflections on their homeland trips reveal two contradictory conceptions of belonging to Vietnam. On the one hand, Vietnam figures as the country to which the children are connected through their relatives. As Tuyet asserts, "Vietnam is my home because my family lives there." Tuyet, who has visited Vietnam only once since coming to the Czech Republic 10 years ago, further stresses in her account, "I miss Vietnam, because my relatives are dying there and I saw them only once in my life and I am afraid I will not remember them at all. I want go there again soon, before they all die." The fear of grandparents' dying is at the same time fear of losing the connection to Vietnam, and to a basic part of the family tree that mediates the connection between the children and Vietnam. The impossibility of being in more intensive touch with Vietnamese relatives because of financial constraints, time requirements, etc.—is articulated with sadness in the voice.

On the other hand, some children who expected to "feel at home" in Vietnam prior to the trip, were disappointed at not feeling that when they actually went there. Many interviewees told me that they "recognized at first sight" that they "did not live in Vietnam." Their homeland trip experiences are similar to those of second-generation Chinese- and Korean-Americans described by Nazli Kibria (2002, p.296), which "highlight to the second generation their marginality or other ways in which they were not accepted and did not belong in Chinese or Korean societies." The experience of being seen as different by the local population (caused by differences in language, dress or demeanor, etc.) was mentioned in all the interviews. This suggests that when talking about Vietnam as the country of their ancestors, children referred exclusively to their kinship genealogy and lineage, as opposed to the country of Vietnam, itself. In other words, it is family genealogy, and not the Vietnamese people as a whole, which represent belonging to the imagined community (Anderson, 1983) of kinship.

Unlike Hanh, who lamented that she had "no home," Tuyet considered both Vietnam and the Czech Republic as her homelands. In the following excerpt she explains why, paying particular attention to the certainties which both countries can provide her.

> Both countries function for me as guarantees of certainty. Here it is the language; the certainty that I can understand here, I understand the new, everything, I think in the Czech language, I have dreams in Czech. And plus my friends and all I have developed here. If I moved to Vietnam, I would have nothing but the family there. In Vietnam I have another kind of certainty; it is the family to which I can always turn to, because it is my family. And Vietnam is my country of birth, the country in the shape of the letter S by the sea. It is just my country, it is difficult to explain. And the Czech Republic, I grew up here.

In Tuyet's account (as in nearly all children's accounts), we can see the dichotomy in understanding homeland and kinship as a relationship based on "existence" versus on "performance." While Vietnam is the homeland because the family is there, the homeland in the Czech Republic is acquired through a process—growing up, learning/speaking the language, making friends, etc. Tuyet's two homes—Vietnam and the Czech Republic—evoke different emotions, memories, and meanings, and provide different frames of reference for belonging and future life trajectories.

6.1.3 Trai: Knowing and Feeling of Belonging

Trai came to the Czech Republic at the age of seven, and his parents immediately found him a nanny to pick him up from kindergarten (where he had to go because of a lack of Czech proficiency) and later from school. He does not remember having a close relationship with his nanny at that early point, as he and his family soon moved away to another part of the Czech Republic, and lost touch with his nanny for several years. Then, when Trai's younger sister was one year old, she began living at the nanny's home, and Trai began spending the summer holidays there, too. Trai addressed his sister's nanny as "grandma" or "Grandma Jindřiška," and recalled many activities he did with her or thanks to her. Like other children, he said "I had a beautiful childhood," and recounted memories of walking in the forest, making campfires, baking potatoes in the fire, going fishing, etc. When I asked Trai what the term "grandmother" meant to him, and who was his grandmother, he replied without hesitation:

> Trai: I have never thought about it, I know that I had my grandmothers, the mother of my mother and of my father.
>
> Adéla: And what is the difference between your grandma, the mother's mother, and Grandma Jindřiška?
>
> Trai: I have no illusions that Grandma Jindřiška would be only my grandma. And I know who my real grandma is, although I do not have as strong ties with her as I have with my Czech granny. But I know where I belong and I know which grandma is my blood grandma and which is my emotional grandma.

This excerpt makes evident the differences in Trai's perception of his ties to his Vietnamese grandmother versus his ties to his Czech grandmother. Like Hanh, Trai distinguishes between "blood" and "emotion." The emotions are generated through activities done together. As Trai says, "Grandma Jindřiška gave us a family life and home that our parents could not provide us." Yet at the same time, Trai does not hesitate to refer to his Vietnamese grandmother as his *only* grandmother, even though his emotional ties with her are much weaker than with his Czech grandmother. Most importantly, he answers this question by saying "I *know* where I belong." Contrary to Hanh and Tuyet who construct their belonging on the emotional basis ("feel warmth of home," "feel safe" etc.), when Trai seeks for the roots of his belonging, he uses rather rational explanations which gives him solid ground under his feet. While Hanh's transnational ties are not *yet* developed, Tuyet is *already* establishing those ties, and Trai has *never* doubted their existence and strength. This is why he emphasizes a strict line between Czech Republic and Vietnam. It is apparent not only from the vocabulary he uses—"blood grandma" versus "emotional grandma"—but from the entire rhetoric he employs when contrasting these two modes of kinship ties. In his account, Trai stresses the importance of his Czech grandmother in his family life and childhood in the earlier years of his life. At this later stage of his life, however, Trai minimizes the role of his Czech grandmother, and instead places importance on other family/kinship ties that that lead him to prefer his Vietnamese grandparents.

There are three factors in his gradual realization of where he belongs. The *first* factor was his trip to Vietnam. After 11 years living in the Czech Republic, Trai, his sister, and his parents decided to visit their relatives in Vietnam. "It was incredibly strong," Trai told me, and described how it was meeting his relatives after such a long time. "It was a shock for all of us" he said, and concluded that this trip—to which he referred as "a holiday"—"renewed" his bond with Vietnam. What exactly was renewed? In Trai's case, it was above all the realization of his place in the kinship network and family hierarchy, and the acceptance of his position as the offspring of Vietnamese ancestors.

The *second* formative factor is Trai's position in the "traditional" Vietnamese family hierarchy. As the son of his grandparents' oldest son, Trai is the bearer of many privileges and responsibilities in both his immediate family and that of his father. It is Trai who is sole heir of his father's parents, the one who can sit at the table with his grandfather while others have to sit on the floor when eating dinner. The responsibilities that Trai's father has (and Trai later will have) include sending remittances to the grandmother, who "lives only on what we send her." Trai knows that this will be expected of him, and that later, when his parents return to Vietnam, he will be expected to provide for them as well (see Kibria, 1993, p.131–132). Trai expressed many times his appreciation and respect for this family system, and declared his will to be part of it. Acceptance of this position made him re-think his relations with his parents. "I missed the family ties and time spent together with my parents when I was younger," he told me. "But now I am really grateful for everything they have done for me and I understand why they could not give me their attention," he confessed. His remarks were filled with great respect, similar to that articulated by several other interviewees (see Chapter 5).

The *third* formative factor in Trai's feeling of belonging are the changes in his conceptions of a "life partner," his ideas about future family life, and his anticipated role as father. Because of the age of my interviewees, the issue of life partners was echoed often in the interviews. Vietnamese parents were regarded as more conservative than Czech parents on this issue, and less open to teenage dating or unmarried cohabitation. In Trai's account, there was a big emphasis put on his change of preference from Czech girlfriends to *the* Vietnamese girlfriend. "Until recently I did not know where I belonged, and I had relationships with Czech girls," Trai told me, and then described to me how he had returned to his Vietnamese heritage and traditions.

If the cases of Hanh and Tuyet illuminate the importance of *backward* continuity, Trai's case sheds light on the equal importance of forward continuity. We can observe stress on the backward continuity in the narratives where the issue of ancestor is very important for developing the sense of belonging to a particular unit—kinship or nation state—from which the heritage can be transmitted to an individual. Forward continuity is manifested in the emphasis on the future generation(s) and the heritage the person can transmit—i.e. ensuring the continuation of Vietnamese traditions, and above all the model of family ties, which Trai describes as typically Vietnamese. The desire for forward continuity may be particularly marked in Trai's case, due to his age and position in the family system. It may also be due to Trai's repeatedly failed relationships with Czech girlfriends. Trai told me that he used to have very nice Czech girlfriends, but that the relationships always ended at the moment they wanted to introduce each other to their respective parents. It simply never happened, as "none of us was able to defend the relationship." Trai then met his current girlfriend, an event that fundamentally changed his understanding of who he is. "Since last year I have had a Vietnamese girlfriend, who has opened my eyes and shown me what bonds are between families; the bond there is just stronger," said Trai. He stressed that having a Vietnamese girlfriend and wife was the best possible choice for him, as in the future he wants to perpetuate his parents' heritage.

6.2 The Czech Republic is My Brain, Vietnam is My Heart

Despite the diversity of these three case studies and accounts, there are some basic similarities among them. The three case studies have illuminated the importance of kinship ties and family norms in the children's formation of a sense of belonging. Put simply, the basic finding of the analysis is: My *homeland is where my family is*. Kinning the Vietnamese relatives in Vietnam is hence an inherent part of establishing feelings of belonging. As the case studies make clear, transnational kinship negotiations vary among interviewees. While Hanh's transnational ties are not *yet* developed, Tuyet is *already* establishing those ties, and Trai has *never* doubted their existence and strength.

In this section, I will first summarize how the issue of family ties is understood in the imagination of homeland (6.2.1). Then I will make an argument that while children of Vietnamese parents brought up by Czech grandmothers are continually oscillating between two conceptions of kinship ties, these children are also wavering back and forth between different notions of belonging (6.2.2). Last but not least, I will briefly conclude with how child interviewees imagine their future relationship with what they now imagine as the homeland (6.2.3). As will be elaborated further, all of these issues are reflected in the metaphor adopted by one of interviewees to express his divided feelings for the Czech Republic and Vietnam; "the Czech Republic is my brain, Vietnam is my heart."

6.2.1 The Strength of Family Ties and Intergenerational Solidarity

It is not surprising that the family is one of the main points of reference for the children I interviewed. Both the family life provided by the Czech grandmother and nuclear family—children and parents—along with its overlap with relatives in Vietnam, were frequently mentioned by child interviewees. It also came up often when I asked about the differences between "Czech" and "Vietnamese upbringings" (see Chapter 4). Concurrent with the findings of Nazli Kibria (1993, p.9), child interviewees appreciated "the traditional Vietnamese family system for its ethic of collectivism and cooperation," and contrasted it with what they considered the selfishness and individualism of Czech society. When asked "what makes you Vietnamese," and the consequence of their Vietnamese upbringing, children commonly responded "I have respect for my family." When asked "Who are you?" or "Where do you belong?," interviewees typically referred to their family, and to the importance of having three generations: grandparents, parents, and partners.

As pointed out previously, *grandparents* and their position in the family genealogy and hierarchy are important links in connecting children to their genealogy and to Vietnam. The Vietnamese tradition of according authority and respect on the basis of seniority (at the core of the traditional family system) makes grandchildren responsible for the well-being of their ancestors. Trai's understanding and acceptance of his family responsibilities (as part of intergenerational family solidarity), and of his position in the family hierarchy, redefined his sense of belonging to a kinship unit and to Vietnam. If the children were looking for a solid point from which to understand their place in the world, this family hierarchy—together with the obligations and responsibilities inherent in it—offered it to them, even if only at a distance.

So far *the parents* have been presented in this chapter as the mediators between children and grandparents. It would of course be misleading to minimize their role as channels between generations. It is above all the parents who pass on the cultural memory of Vietnam to their children. Besides language, their personal stories from the Vietnam War were mentioned as formative events for their children. Some nannies (such as Ms. Zezulková, Ms. Havranová, and so on) marveled at how the parents were able to "foster such a strong national feeling for Vietnam" (as Ms. Zezulková puts it) when they were with the children only a few hours a day. At the same time, there are intangible and unspoken messages to which the children are very sensitive, and which give them a clear message that only Vietnam is their parents' home, while the Czech Republic is merely a place of work (as already discussed in Chapter 3). "I love my mum, and my dad is a life-long paragon for me," Lien, a 17-year-old girl told me when I asked her to tell me something about her parents. Like other children I interviewed, Lien referred to her parents' diligence and self-sacrifice, which always impressed her. Her parents were her source of love and respect. Child interviewees commonly pointed to the hard life of their parents in the Czech Republic, and to the fact that such an intensive work life did not allow their parents the opportunity to make friends or have fun. This difficult life in the Czech Republic was contrasted with what children observed during their visits to Vietnam. As Yen sadly described:

> After my dad passed away, my mum saved up money for a trip to Vietnam. When we got there, it was the first time I saw my mum really happy. My mum is a huge optimist, which I do not understand at all. Sometimes I am not nice to her, yet she is smiling all the time. She went through tough times, and when she returned to Vietnam for couple of days, I could see how happy she was there. It was only one month and ten days or something like that. And then she came back to reality and started to work and work again.

Visiting Vietnam showed these children where the home of their parents was, and how their own feelings about belonging resembled and differed from those of their parents. At the same time, this visit to Vietnam made children realize that in a few years, they, too, would be going to Vietnam to see their parents.

Last but not least, there are *future families and current partners*, who shape children's aspirations and expectations for future relations. Trai's account suggests that the continuity that my interviewees seek is directed not only towards the "imagined past," but also towards a "planned future." The choice of a life partner and friends is critical here. While for Trai the only possible choice is a Vietnamese girlfriend, many of my interviewees leave this decision open to "what the heart says." It would be misleading to expect that only Vietnamese partners can foster "Vietnameseness." The contrary happened, for instance, in the case of Thi. Like other interviewees in my sample, Thi had adopted a Czech name—in her case, Eliška—as it made her feel more comfortable with her peers and friends. However, one day her Czech boyfriend called her by her Vietnamese name "Thi," and from then on she started introducing herself as Thi, as a manifestation of her origins, as she described it.

There is no evidence among child interviewees of systematic preference for endogamy or exogamy. Their parents, on the other hand, would prefer that their children found Vietnamese partners—as they feel it would be more practical (because of the language barriers) and useful for the future (maintenance of family tradition). However, Vietnamese parents said they were most concerned that their children be happy and not feel pushed into anything in that regard.

6.2.2 Naturalization of Homeland and Socialization through Homeland

What points of reference do the children have at their disposal in order to "belong" to Vietnam? It is not the language, as many of them (not all of them, of course) do not speak fluent Vietnamese, and consider Czech as their first language. Only some of them can cite birthplace as the foundation of their ties to Vietnam. Only a few have a personal history and memories of childhood spent there. Eventually, kinship may provide them with a sense of belonging. However, as Chapter 5 has demonstrated, even the idea of kinship is highly ambiguous, and does not serve as the children's *sole* frame of reference. Instead there are two frames of reference, each of which is experienced and defined differently. The imagination of homeland through kinship ties is unclear for the grandchildren of Vietnamese grandmothers who are brought up by Czech grandmothers. When speaking about kinship and belonging, children draw upon two emic definitions: a primordial (biogenetic) one in the case of Vietnam, and a constructivist (performative) one in the case of the Czech Republic.

Negotiation of belonging takes place on the symbolic borders between culture and nature, as it is "structured around the reference to the naturalness of the idea of origin, ancestors (…) or the myth of common blood" (Šlesingerová, 2005, p.116). The ideas of blood and genes pervade interviewees' accounts. At a time when an awareness of genomics is growing, popular discourse is filled with references to the connection between genes and the idea of origin, national identity, etc. (Šlesingerová, 2014). These ideas become important for second-generation children, for whom the "naturalness" of belonging in the Czech Republic is challenged by the people around them, by their parents, and by themselves. As Tuyet told me, "I am different, I look different so I cannot put aside my Vietnamese origin; I cannot struggle against being seen as different. And why should I?" The idea of primordial membership rooted in the symbolism of blood and genes offers them a concept of belonging with enduring significance (Kibria, 2002). According to Kibria (2002, p.303), notions of a primordial identity provide second- generation Chinese and Korean Americans "an important counterpoint to the uncertainties they felt about their membership and belonging as Chinese or Korean." Likewise, Yen Le Espiritu (2003) emphasizes that many migrants articulate their sense of home by overemphasizing ties of biology and geography.

As Kibria (2002, p.303) points out, it is not surprising that second- generation immigrants see personal belonging derived from a "primordial" notion of identity as more "authentic" and "true" than a "circumstantial and artificial" sense of belonging due to "an accident of migration." This was very much visible in the story of Hanh, for whom the outcomes of her parents' migration were one of the main issues in her accounts of belonging and kinship. This distinction between authentic and artificial is further imprinted in the way the homeland is narrated and imagined. I would argue that the accounts reveal the children's dual notion of homeland—a place based on genetics, blood and family on the one hand in the case of Vietnam and, on the other hand, a place of social relationships in the case of the Czech Republic. These two simultaneous processes are apparent in Hanh's account, which is built upon the difference between the home that was taken from them by their parents, and the home that was created for them by their Czech grandmother. It also appears in Tuyet's perception of home that exists thanks to the family in Vietnam, and the home that she herself has actively created when living in the Czech Republic.

The children's active role in *developing* ties with the Czech Republic contrasts with the fairly passive and "taken-for-granted" existence of Vietnam with which ties *already* exist, and that are awakened by the practices of emotional transnationalism. The Czech Republic is located on the children's mental map as the country where they grew up and attended school; it is the place where they have their friends and Czech grandmothers that introduced them, and helped them adapt to Czech culture and society (see above).

Balancing between two homelands and upbringings, some children refer to themselves as "banana kids" as a way of describing the ambiguity of their identity and sense of belonging. "We are yellow (Vietnamese) on the surface but white (Czech) on the inside." In adopting this metaphor to describe themselves, these children portray both the strength of their origins ("I am from Vietnam because I look like Vietnamese") as well as the importance of their upbringing ("I am Czech because I think like a Czech"). Some children, on the other hand, reject the "banana kid" concept, as they do not feel themselves truly Czech, even "on the inside." As Tuyet explained:

> Vietnamese kids are not purely white inside, they always have the Vietnamese core, it is just there, even though they do not admit it. And as they grow up, at the age of 18 or 19, there is a break in their life. And the child starts realizing that she has some roots and starts being interested in her culture and everything.

In line with what has been covered in this chapter, Tuyet's account rests upon the indisputable existence of Vietnamese roots that cannot be denied. Sooner or later these roots will come to the fore, when children reflect on their belonging and the imagination of homeland. "We are the children of our Vietnamese parents," many interviewees told me. However, the question remains as to how these children will refer to themselves later on, when they start their own families. Will they be Vietnamese parents for their children? And what will they tell the children about their roots and where they belong?

In summary, the interviewees' accounts contain two stories about belonging and kinship ties. The first story is about the connection with the Czech grandmother and the Czech Republic, and is based on the leitmotif of memories, acquired relationships, and overall assimilation to life in the Czech Republic (above all in the social and cultural capital). The second story is about Vietnamese relatives and Vietnam, and is inspired by the desire to belong to something enduring, unchangeable and corporeal (based on blood and genes). This story provides the meta-narrative of belonging that starts in the family and transforms into belonging to the imagined community of the nation state.

6.2.3 Transforming Homeland into "Holidayland"

The stories of Hanh, Tuyet and Trai show that even though Vietnam is imagined as a homeland, none of the children actually imagines returning there to live. What kind of relationships do they want to maintain with Vietnam? And what kind of relations do they wish to maintain with the Czech Republic?

As I discussed above, trips to Vietnam are interpreted by my interviewees as turning points in their lives. However, despite the fact that for many children the trip to Vietnam meant a "return to their roots," their notion of "return" has two meanings here. First is the concept of returning in the sense of "turning back" and finding one's roots. Second is the idea of returning in the sense of "going there at times" to see family and spend the holidays. The average number of Vietnam visits made by interviewees was around two visits in their entire life or since coming to the Czech Republic. One of my interviewees, Khanh, told me she wanted to spend one year in Vietnam after she finishing her university studies in order to see what life was like there. Another interviewee, Lien, said she did not want to visit Vietnam very often so that Vietnam did not become "ordinary" to her. Vietnam, therefore, figures in the accounts as an imagined homeland in an imagined past, and as a "holidayland" in an imagined future. This future plan was largely shaped by their experience of marginalization in Vietnam. Thi, who lived in Vietnam until the age of 5, describes her three visits to Vietnam as follows:

"I was like a tourist in my own country. I still take Vietnam as an important part of my life. It is something from my past, but it is not finished; the relationship still persists in myself, in my interaction with people, with my family." It is the need to continue the relationship with Vietnam, combined with the feeling of both belonging there ("my own country") and not belonging ("I was like a tourist") that is apparent in Thi's account. This ambivalence—which appears in many other interviews—shapes children's ties with Vietnam. While the children maintain strong emotional ties with Vietnam, these ties are not strong enough to motivate children to "give up the life in Europe" in which they have grown up.

When it comes to the Czech Republic as a homeland, the visions of interviewees are far from uniform. While some children plan to move to Western countries (the United Kingdom, France or the USA figure here as the dream destinations), others cannot imagine leaving the Czech Republic, and declare themselves loyal Czech patriots, who love the Czech culture and language (such as Tuyet or Linh). In almost all cases the Czech Republic figures in their future plans as the "country where I want to be returning" after trips and stays abroad in Western Europe or the US. Their reasons for returning will not be parents (who will most likely have returned to Vietnam), but rather siblings, friends, and their imagined future families. In summary, the Czech Republic will be the homeland to which they return after visiting their relatives in their other homeland, Vietnam.

* * *

The previous section on kinning looked at how children are kinned to their nannies' grandchildren, and how nannies are kinned to the grandmothers of cared-for children. This section examined the similar process of home-bonding. While the previous section pointed out the ambiguities in kinship definitions, this section analyzed how these ambiguities are reflected and even strengthened in the imaginative process of homeland creation. Interviewees have "blood grandmothers" and "emotional grandmothers," as Trai describes it; they have "blood family" and "soul family," as Hanh puts it; and they have their "heart in Vietnam" and "brain in the Czech Republic," as Hue states it. Such language appears repeatedly in my interviews with child interviewees, and reflects the basic tensions of belonging. As the question of "where do I belong" is usually answered by reference to the family or kinship, children that experience tension between the two modes of kinship also experience tension in belonging to two imagined communities.

6.4 Provisional Conclusions to Chapter 5 and Chapter 6: The Accounts of Kinning and Belonging

Chapter 5 has examined mutual dependency in nanny-child relationships by focusing on the issue of care-giving as a principal practice of kinning, during which the children are assigned the role of grandchildren, and nannies the role of grandmothers. As a consequence of separation from actual blood kin, Czech nannies commonly supplant Vietnamese grandmothers, while cared for children in turn often supplant nannies' own or missing biological children and/or grandchildren. Some women become nannies due to missing intergenerational ties with blood family, which they try to replace by caring for other people's children.

This chapter compared similarities between accounts of kinship and accounts of belonging. The statement "Home is where my family is" is inherently unclear when the definitions of "family" and "home" are themselves ambiguous. Throughout this chapter, I have attempted to answer the question of how second-generation Vietnamese children brought-up by Czech nannies conceive of kinship and homeland. The answer can be found in Figure 6.1, which presents the main issues addressed in this chapter, and illustrates how homeland is defined by kinship, which is based on biogenetic and social relatedness.

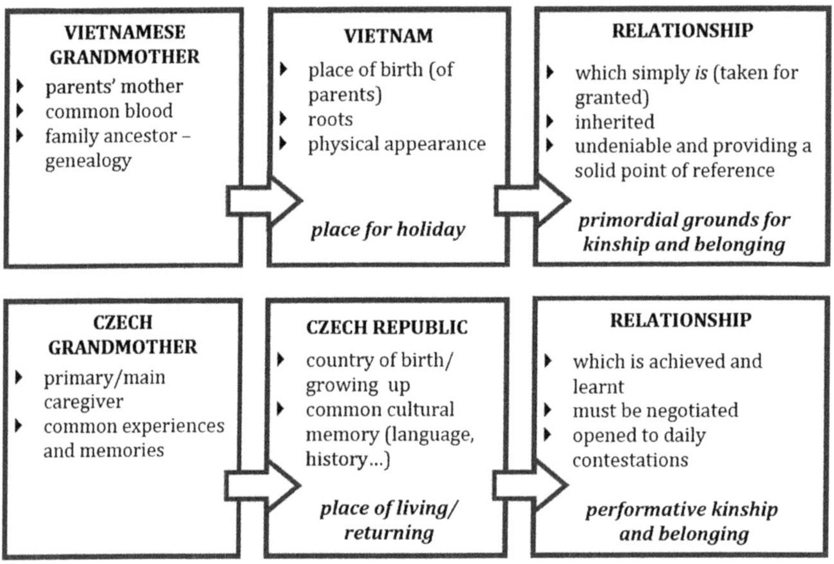

Figure 6.1 Parallels between accounts of kinship/homeland belonging

This figure provides a guide to a dual understanding of the relationship between the narrative of kinship and the narrative of belonging. First, the figure can be read as "kinship shapes the belonging to the imagined community of the nation state." The story of "belonging through kinship" is that Czech grandmothers provide their Vietnamese grandchildren with a Czech home and family life (through the daily performance of care-giving), and help them to understand and experience Czech traditions; hence Czech grandmothers are important actors in establishing a sense of belonging. Vietnamese grandmothers, on the other hand, provide grandchildren with the story of common blood and ancestry, and link children with their place in the family genealogy; hence the Vietnamese grandmothers connect children to their roots in Vietnam.

Second, the figure can be read as the "intra-action of the narrative of kinship and narrative of belonging." The two narratives share the same rhetoric—employing similar vocabulary, metaphors, and symbols. When speaking about Vietnam, children use the same vocabulary as when they speak about their Vietnamese grandmothers. The same holds true when children speak about the Czech Republic—their words are similar to those used when speaking of their Czech grandmothers. The children simply *have* their Vietnamese grandmothers, with whom the relationship is based on common blood and shared genes. One of the homelands *is* Vietnam, because they have their roots there. But the children I interviewed *establish* ties with their Czech grandmothers—they are brought up by them and share their memories. These children also *develop* ties to the Czech Republic by growing up in the country and learning the Czech language and way of life. As the case studies presented in Chapter 6 clearly demonstrated, children are active in constructing their ties both with Czech grandmothers and the Czech Republic, and to Vietnamese grandmothers and Vietnam—the kinship ties as well as one's feeling of belonging require great "agency work" and negotiations in developing and creating what can be later perceived as taken-for granted and/or explained in terms of blood and biological relatedness. Such "agency work" is recognized by children when it comes to belonging to the Czech Republic, and having kinship ties with Czech grandmothers both of which appear in the interviews as negotiated, requiring the children's agency—and as such they are always open to redefinitions. Contrary to the image of the Czech Republic with which the relationship must be re-negotiated every day, the level of agency is made invisible in the case of Vietnam which, as a homeland, is paradoxically, stable, unchangeable and indisputable, despite the fact that children visit it very rarely.

Chapter 7
Conclusion: Mutual Dependency, Emotionality, and Kinship Ties in Care-Giving

"Migration uproots, and replanting takes time," wrote Charles Tilly and C. Harold Brown in 1967 (Tilly and Brown, 1967, p.139). After coming to the Czech Republic and starting families here, Vietnamese parents deal with how to replant their child care and family ideologies in a new context. While being part of a transnational social field enables them to keep in touch with mothering strategies in Vietnam (through their relatives or friends, by following the situation there, etc.), living in the Czech Republic throws them into a different setting where different *normal caring biographies* are supported. Changes in family structure after migration (intensification of work life at the expense of family life and uprooting from extensive kinship networks that care can be delegated to) lead families to find a "substitute" grandmother for their children—a Czech nanny. Having a Czech nanny is becoming the post-migration norm in the Vietnamese community. While only 1–2 percent of Czech families make use of individual private paid child care, my interviewees estimated that the number of Vietnamese families seeking nannies for their children is around 80–95 percent. Most of them add that this is a "common," "normal," or "matter-of-fact" thing. In addition, it is not only "common" to have a nanny, it is also "normal" that strong (even permanent) ties between the nanny and the children emerge.

Research on Vietnamese immigrant families hiring Czech nannies in the Czech Republic has attempted to reveal the character of mutual dependencies in childcare work. The first step towards portraying the complex dynamics of delegated care-giving was incorporating children into the research agenda. Interviews with now adult children (aged 16 to 25 years) spoke about their experiences with nannies and mothers illuminated several essential aspects of care work: its emotionality, and its role in creating long-lasting bonds. These aspects are barely visible when research is done only with nannies and mothers. Children are not mute and passive recipients of care-giving. They are active agents, with their own ideas and ideals about parents' parenthood and their childhood which they struggle to impose on parents and change their parents' parenting role.

The analysis of immigrant families hiring native nannies can be read as another case study of care-giving work. It can also be read as a case study which—thanks to reversed ethnic logic—brings a new angle to existing scholarship. And above all, it can be read as a case study which—thanks to its specificity within the context of mainstream scholarship—makes visible new issues and aspects of delegated care-giving which are less apparent when immigrant nannies work in non-migrant families. In this book, these new issues were analyzed through the prism of mutual dependency. At the beginning of the research, I asked the main question of *"What is the character of the relationships among mothers, nannies and children?"* In what follows, I will answer this question by distinguishing five characteristics of the relationships in the mother-child-nanny triangle. There are five kinds of mutual dependency, which were analyzed in the book. Some of them could be generally applicable to experiences of care workers, their employers, and cared-for children, while others would be more typical for the immigrant employers (both those with immigrant care workers and native care workers).

Mutual Economic Dependency and Relationships Based on *Paid* Care-Giving

On a basic level, there is always the *employment* relationship between employers (mothers) and employees (nannies), between a woman who pays and a woman who is paid. On the demand side are families who can afford to pay the nannies, and on the supply side are the nannies for whom paid care-giving is a breadwinning activity and often the main source of income. That is why care work is analyzed as reflecting, generating, and reproducing class inequalities among women, and as being a base for gendered class relations (Momsen, 1999). Having a nanny or domestic worker has been described as *a marker of social status*, the privilege of middle- or upper-class families. At the same time, being a nanny or domestic worker has been considered a sign of lower class (Momsen, 1999; Gregson and Lowe, 1994). As many scholars argue, domestic work relationships not only mirror already-existing class inequalities, but generate new class relation constellations that need to be described with new conceptual terms. For example Gregson and Lowe (1994), in their analysis of the British domestic work experience, established a distinction between the "new middle class" (demand) and the "servant class" (supply of care/domestic work). Apparently, these two groups are mutually constructed and do not exist a priori. Class distinctions are not limited to merely material possessions, but also extend to "the privilege of having constant caring and nurturing" (Romero, 1997, p.161) and they originate in the fact that "one is selling her labour to the other for a wage" (Stiell and England, 1997, p.342). It can therefore be concluded that one is not born a member of the servant class, but rather becomes one.

Gregson and Lowe (1994) admit that some nannies (more often than housekeepers) may be from middle-class families, and that one needs to look at the nannies' socio-economic position in their country of origin (Parreñas, 2001; Lutz, 2011; Yeates, 2009). When so doing, we can see that for some women migration for domestic work is not merely a survival strategy, but a matter of maintaining a certain social status and lifestyle (Lutz, 2011). To capture the nature of the class status of migrant domestic workers, Parreñas (2001) comes up with the notion of "contradictory class mobility." She uses this term to refer to the simultaneous experience of upward and downward mobility in the migration of domestic workers which causes both an increase in financial status and a decline in social status. While these studies challenge the image of domestic workers as poor members of the working class, they do not address the assumption that demanders of paid care or domestic work are rich families. In other words, the marker of "middle-class" remains central for the description of employers.

In the 1990s, scholars of black feminism began to point out deficiencies in the conceptualization of motherhood, which they considered class-biased and Western-centric, and blind to the experiences of working class women and non-western ethnicities (see Glenn, 994). I dare say that this is also the case with the conceptualization of domestic work, which is also class-biased and Western-centric. Domestic work is typically defined through the experience of the (white) middle classes of the Western world, who demand services usually provided by immigrant women. Paradoxically, while criticizing the middle-class definition of motherhood, feminist scholars have been producing a middle-class definition of care work. As the case study of immigrant families hiring native nannies shows, paid care work in households need not be a middle-class privilege, but also a necessity for a lower class for which a dual income is indispensable.

This is not to say that all the families I contacted were from a lower social class. In this regard my sample is quite varied—it includes cases of rich families as well as families whose economic conditions are poorer than those of the nannies. For all these families the delegation of care-giving subsequently leads to upward mobility:—the parents can focus solely on earning money, which can be used for promoting the children's upward mobility through their education. Despite the diversity within my sample, the mother-interviewees were univocal in emphasizing the economic necessity of having a nanny (paying her a very low wage), in order to allow the parents to participate in breadwinning activities. For Vietnamese mothers, the need for a nanny originates in their efforts to fulfil the financially burdensome definition of motherhood in the post-migratory context, and is not a mark of the family's socio-economic status. Consequently, the privilege and mark of a higher socio-economic position would be to *not* have a nanny, but rather to be an a stay at home mother, and wife of a man earning so much that the family does not need a second breadwinner.

At the same time, when it comes to the nannies, none of them work as nannies *just* for the money, and some do not work because of the money at all. Considering the typical monthly salary of a nanny—which on average does not even reach the minimum wage in the Czech Republic—the motivations to become nannies must be sought in the context of the nannies' (caring) biographies and not solely by looking at their family budget. Hence, when addressing mutual economic dependence, Czech nannies in Vietnamese families provide us an alternative understanding of paid care-giving. For nannies, the salary for care-giving does not provide their main income, as all of them have income from social benefits. It means that when entering this line of work, for some nannies the salary means a financial contribution to the budget, while for other nannies the money is irrelevant to their decision.

The mutual economic dependency between Vietnamese mothers and Czech nannies is not the most important aspect of their ties; it is just one piece of the puzzle, which together with other kinds of dependencies, paints the full picture of the relationships between mothers, children, and nannies. In the case of nannies, economic dependency is weakened when the emotional and intergenerational dependencies are established. For mothers, the economic dependency is the means for accomplishing the ideal of good motherhood and creating the mutual dependency in motherhood definitions between themselves and nannies.

Mutual Emotional Dependency and the Definition of Paid Care-Giving

Following the first layer of mutual dependency and the analysis of the motivations to become a nanny, the second characteristic of the mother-nanny-child triangular relationship leads us inevitably to the emotionality of care-giving. Care-giving work is inherently an emotional activity that requires and generates emotional attachment and investment. The emotional attachment exhibited by nannies' toward cared-for children was described by several researchers (Nelson, 1990; Macdonald, 1998). However, no one has yet addressed how the children respond to such attachment and what their attitudes to nannies are. Once again we see the importance of incorporating children into the research agenda in order to fully understand the role and nature of emotional attachment. The accounts of nannies and children show that one of the main characteristics of their ties is that they are based on mutual emotional exchange.

Analysis of the children's accounts of emotions and emotionality in care work illuminates how children perceive differences in care-giving strategies, and the outcomes of the delegated childcare. Children do not understand the emotions as inevitable, automatic aspects of their ties with nannies and parents. Rather, the children stressed that emotions are generated only in the practice of care-giving—and do not exist a priori because of the biological bonds. The interview with Linh, a 19-year-old girl, shows the differences in children's perception of their relations with parents and nannies: "I felt like they [her parents] were hurting me and I did not understand why they were so cold to me. When I lived with my grandma and grandpa [the nanny and her husband], they kept on clearly showing me their love." The children get from nannies something which they cannot get from their parents—either because the parents are busy with breadwinning activities or because it is not part of parents' definition of parenthood. The emotional exchange children experience with nannies is therefore distinctly different from that experienced with parents. However, this does not mean that children think that there is love missing between themselves and parents. Rather, it means that the love is manifested in a different way—as 17-year old Lien makes evident:

> Normally I do not hug my mum. I have never told her "mum, I love you." But I love her very much of course. She does so much for me and this way she compensate it—even though she does not show it physically or verbally. She shows it when caring about me, providing me with money for anything I want and especially for my education. And that is the compensation for her not saying "I love you."

From the vocabulary that Lien selects to describe her mother's behavior to her ("compensation"), it seems that Lien probably misses the manifestation of emotions, and knows that there is another model of emotional exchange common in Czech families. Both Lien's and Linh's accounts make apparent that while being subjected to two different types of care-giving, the children also experience different kinds of the expression of emotionality. They would probably prefer the emotional exchange they have with their nannies to the emotional "coldness" experienced with their mothers. However, at the same time they know that both types of emotional expression are mutually constructed. The nannies can provide them with hugs, kisses, and presence because the mothers leave for work and provide nannies the time and space for it. At the same time, the nannies are freed from the responsibility of providing children financially, and can therefore provide for the children's emotional needs.

The nannies highlighted in the interviews that care work is an activity which can (and must) be done only when the care worker likes children—either in general, or at least the child in particular that the nanny is caring for. As Chapter 3 showed, an emotional investment is necessary for becoming a nanny. Common motivations are the "need to be needed," the "desire for a meaningful hobby," or the "doing activity which I like performing," etc. These needs and desires are met in the daily practice of care-giving for a Vietnamese child– and then the emotional investment shifts into the emotional satisfaction. Mutual emotional exchange is therefore more than a by-product of care-giving. For many nannies, this emotional exchange is the *raison d'être* of their care-giving—from the decision to become a nanny, to the daily performance of tasks which are paid far below labour market standards. That is why the nannies define both care-giving and their role of nannies through the acknowledgement of emotional ties with the children, and not through their employment relations with the mothers/parents (see below).

Between nannies and children, emotions flow both ways. Emotional investment does not imply that the nanny is actively passing her feelings on to child, who is only a passive recipient. Emotions manifest themselves in a form of a gift which entails giving, receiving and reciprocating (Mauss, 1922). All the attention and affection which the nanny passes to a child returns back to her—in the form of making her feel loved and needed. This logic of the two-way channel of affection is apparent in the statement by Ms. Dudková, who talks about her ties with her Vietnamese granddaughter: "I love her and she gives me everything back." This nanny, as well as others, was afraid of losing the touch with the child. The end of care-giving—either caused by the independence of the child or by the parents' decision—was a painful issue in the interviews with nannies. The end of care-giving meant not only the end of a breadwinning activity, but of an activity that brought emotional satisfaction to the nanny's life. Consequently, the great importance of emotionality in care-giving work impacts on how nannies relate to their role as nannies and how they define their position *vis-à-vis* mothers.

Compared to the warm feelings exchanged between nannies and children, ties between nannies and mothers are rather distant. The nannies and mothers have few opportunities to develop a relationship based on mutual understanding because of the lack of communication. Mothers and nannies do not spend much time together and even if they do, they encounter a language barrier. The mothers usually welcome the fact that the nannies love the children in their care. The mothers are persuaded that the nanny will never replace the mothers' role, especially in those cases where the care contract was established between three generations. When the nanny is at the age of mother's mother—and hence like the child's grandmother—the mother normally feels that her exclusive place in child's life is secure. In cases where the age difference between mother and nanny is not significant, and the nanny may be possibly viewed as the child's "aunt"—the mother's exclusive place may be potentially challenged. However, the mothers did not express any worries about weakening their ties with children as a consequence of care-giving delegation, or of their children developing emotional ties with nannies. This certainty about mothers' unquestionable and stable position in children's lives stems from the mothers' definition of good motherhood and of family (see below).

If the key term characterizing the nanny-child relationship is "emotional satisfaction," in nanny-mother ties the key term is "emotional recognition." Care-giving becomes a part of nannies' lives, of their gendered biographies (see below), and the nannies' claims for recognition are formulated in this spirit. It is their emotional investment in the children, the quality of care which they provide them, and the skills which they pass on to them which must be recognized and valued—especially by mothers. Many nannies say in describing their role in the lives of cared for children, "We taught them everything," and contrast their emotional involvement in the children's wellbeing to that of the mothers. The nannies thus do not measure their self-worth in terms of wages, but rather in terms of their critical role (or even primacy) in care-giving and in shaping the personalities of the children. The absence of this recognition would be experienced as a threat to their gendered biographies—not "only" as a failure to perform their job tasks. The nannies therefore do not feel exploited when they reflect on their salary or work conditions. However they *do* feel exploited when mothers do not recognize the importance of the nanny in the child's life. Failure to recognize the nanny's role is viewed by the nannies as a demonstration of unequal power relations in which the nannies always (sooner or later) lose. Despite the nannies' strong emotional ties with the children, the nannies are aware that their care-giving can be terminated anytime because they are not the children's biological mothers.

Mutual Dependency in Care-Giving Strategies in Definitions of Motherhood and Womanhood

The relationship between employer and employee is a relationship between two women, both of whom enter the relationship with their own ideas, ideals, and experience of motherhood. These—very often clashing—ideas are further reproduced and even strengthened during daily care-giving, and create a climate in which the mother-nanny relationship is negotiated. Mutual dependency in motherhood means that paid care-giving enables mothers and nannies to do motherhood—and what they consider to be "good motherhood"—according to their own scenario. This scenario is based on their differing resources and performed at the intersections of differing cultural, social, and economic worlds. At the same time, because motherhood is shaped as the expression of women's natural identity (McMahon, 1995), the delegation of care-giving becomes an arena for mutual negotiations of womanhood definitions and gender identity work.

For Vietnamese mothers in my sample, mothering is realized through participation in the labour market and its main aim is to provide "a better tomorrow" for second generation children. In this regard, the mothers' testimonies contribute to scholarship that seeks to redefine mothering to include providing for children's financial needs (Erel, 2009). In order to be a "good mother," the mother must dedicate her life to breadwinning activity and look for a nanny. The decision to hire a nanny is therefore a reaction to a post-migratory situation—the shift in work biographies, absence of kin members, and life in a country where different childcare ideals are valid. Under such conditions, the Vietnamese parents create dual-earner households, and transfer performance of their role as parents from the household to the labour market. In other words, doing motherhood requires delegating motherhood. Vietnamese mothers' experiences and reflections show that care-giving and breadwinning dos not have to be in opposition to one another. Rather, breadwinning is a means for providing the supposedly best care-giving possible.

When nannies enter the dual-earner Vietnamese households to take care of Vietnamese children, they experience the clash between their own ideals of motherhood and the strategies employed by the mothers. For nannies, mothering is shaped by physical presence and daily caring for a child. At the same time, nannies understand dedicated (present and at-home) care-giving as the confirmation of their gendered biographies, their womanhood. For nannies that had been full-time mothers, and had spent up to four years with each of their children on parental leave (sacrificing their work biographies to their family life), care-giving is something they have always done, and is a critical activity for their gendered biographies. For nannies that were working mothers with their own children, present care-giving is something they could not do with their own children, but that they need to do now, as it "fills them with energy" and enables them to stay active—both as human beings, and as women by performing the core activity of doing gender. Both former at-home mothers and former working mothers relate paid care-giving to their identities as mothers. While for the former group of women, paid care-giving meant prolonging the active mothering they were at the moment performing, for the latter group, paid care-giving meant additional fulfilment of the intensive mother ideal (which they were unable to experience). And, surprisingly, despite the radically different experiences, the model of intensive, present, and at-home childcare was glorified as the most appropriate arrangement.

All nannies understand care-giving of Vietnamese children as something which they *normally* and *normatively* do. They do it normally in various stages of life (as mothers or grandmothers) when their biographies are defined through the dependence and needs of another person (child, grandchild, husband). And they do it normatively, because they feel they are expected to do it, according to the normative expectations assigned to female subjectivities in the Czech society (embodied for example in the re-familized social policies). If motherhood is represented as "an essential component of her [woman's] identity" (Nelson, 1994, p.182) or "primary responsibilities of adult womanhood" (Macdonald , 2010, p.25) or a core activity of doing gender (Lutz, 2008c), failing as a mother usually means failing as a woman. And for many nannies in my sample, the delegation of mothering—as performed by Vietnamese mothers—is equated with failure. The failure of one means the gain of another—in this case of Czech nannies that can negotiate their gendered subjectivities while taking care of Vietnamese children.

In the context of delegated care-giving, both mothers and nannies mutually construct their images of good motherhood as well as the strategies to fulfil them. Doing motherhood is always an "ongoing interactional accomplishment" (deVault, 1991) in which the identities of mothers and women are shaped. To become a good mother, the Vietnamese mother must provide her children with sufficient economic capital—and she can do so only when the nanny takes care of the children. The mother needs the nanny in order to accomplish her ideas of good mothering. Similarly, the Czech nanny paints her own picture of good motherhood in relation to the mothering strategies of the Vietnamese mother. Equipped with her own experience in mothering, and the further advantage of being Czech and knowing how to raise children well in the Czech Republic, the nanny employs moral hierarchies to judge the mothers' mothering. Doing so, the nanny protects her image of good mothering—which usually means the Czech way of mothering—, and views herself as superior (care-giver) to the Vietnamese mother. In the daily practice of care-giving, mutual dependency means that "what the nanny does, the mother does not have to do." By accepting the job, and the many tasks involved, the nanny allows the mother to not to do these tasks. The care-giving strategies of the mothers are complementary to those of the nannies. These two ways of doing motherhood mutually enable and complement each other, so that the child receives what both mothers and nannies comprehend as the "best care." Despite at times strong criticism directed at Vietnamese mothers, the nannies not only provide "a service in which they do not believe" (Nelson, 1994), but are important actors in the process of creating this service and the demand for it.

Intergenerational Mutual Dependency, Care-Giving and Care-Receiving as the Formative Aspect of Family Relationships

The care work relationship—especially between nannies and children—includes interaction filled with the intimacy, reciprocity, and care that is typical of familial relationships. It is quite common that in making sense of the nanny's place in children's lives, nannies, mothers, and children draw upon the existing codex for family relationships (Murray, 1998; Uttal, 1996). This includes above all the way of addressing each other; the nanny may be called "aunt" or "grandma" to evoke the familial relations. While studies of migrant care workers and au pairs suggest that families create an impression of familial ties in order to exercise "moral economy" and require more work from the care-giver (Hess and Puckhaber, 2004; see also Anderson, 2000; Búriková and Miller, 2010), the Czech nannies I interviewed had radically different experiences. To analyze this experience, the concept of kinning (Howell, 2003) was useful, as it allowed us to reveal the process of becoming relatives. And again, the incorporation of children into the research agenda brought a new perspective on the nature of ties between nannies and children, and between children and parents in the context of delegated care. The case of Vietnamese families and their Czech nannies reveals the critical role of care-giving and care-receiving in the formation of family ties, and exposes another layer of mutual dependency—the dependency in intergenerational relations.

When addressing child-mother relations, the children's accounts indicate the tensions between mothers' and children's understanding of the parent-child relationship. When considering their ties with their parents, child interviewees cited the discrepancy between "they did everything for us" and "they did nothing with us." Children describe their parents as relying on pre-existing child-parent ties that exist simply because the parents are the parents and the children are their children. Contrary to this, the children emphasize the performative aspect of these ties, following the logic of "we must be together and do something together in order to belong to each other." In their view, the ties must be performed in order to exist, and they must generate common memories and the feeling of belonging together—being the daughter/son of mother/father. If this is not so, an intergenerational gap is created that does not allow children to become emotionally closer to their parents and vice versa. This gap—described in terms of emotion, language and mental distance between parents and child—characterizes the situation of many children-interviewees struggling with the dual position of being the child of immigrant parents and being brought up by a person who is not a parent. Their dual position—between a Vietnamese mother and a Czech nanny, between the Czech Republic and Vietnam—fundamentally shapes their ethnic identification and sense of belonging (see socio-cultural mutual dependency below).

Between children and nannies, intensive daily care-giving leads to the establishment of kinship ties. The nannies become grandmothers and children become grandchildren. (The activities necessary for such subjectivation are described in Chapter 5.) The case of Vietnamese children and Czech nannies illuminates the formative role of care-giving as a bonding activity connecting otherwise unconnected people. There does not exist any official confirmation of these ties—such as in the case of adoption which served Howell for developing the notion of kinning. However, the kinship relations are presented both by nannies and by children as ever-lasting and strong enough to be maintained even when the actual need for care-giving is terminated.

Delegated care-giving establishes intergenerational mutual dependency between children (grandchildren) and nannies (grandmothers). This mutual dependency is fostered by the need to experience intergenerational relations and solidarity—to be a grandmother and to be a grandchild. It shows the importance of these relations in older age (in the case of nannies) and during childhood. The base for creating intergenerational kinship ties is the long-term care-giving, which includes reciprocal care-giving and care-receiving. These kinship ties therefore radically differ from those based on biogenetic relatedness. The ties between nannies and children are voluntary—the woman *decides* to become a nanny (her decision is not driven by economic needs) and later *wants* to become a grandmother (and her will is not driven by the biogenetic pre-dispositions).

Kinship ties developed during intensive care-giving provide nannies and children with an arena for self-realization in intergenerational relations, and fulfilment of what they consider the ideals of grandmotherhood and grandchildhood. Thanks to their Vietnamese grandchildren, the Czech nannies can experience the intensive grandmotherhood which they cannot experience with their children's children. Their grandmotherhood with Vietnamese children is much more intensive than is normally the case in Czech society (see Hasmanová Marhánková and Štípková, 2014), and their involvement in childcare exceeds the common standard of grandparental care. For these women, paid care-giving also offers the opportunity to remain active in later life, and helps the women avoid loneliness and boredom after retirement. Intergenerational kinship relations with Czech grandmothers are a source of self-realization for children as well. For the children, their relationship with their Czech grandma—characterized by direct and present engagement—provides an opportunity to experience family life and ties. They can rarely experience family life with their parents, as the parents spend the majority of time in the labour market, engaged in breadwinning activity. And the children's opportunities to experience family life with Vietnamese grandparents are limited because of geographical and personal distance.

Both kinship ties with Czech grandmothers and with relatives in Vietnam require an amount of "kinwork" (di Leonardo, 1987) to develop and be maintained. However, in the children's understanding of kinship, these ties are presented as radically different from one another in regard to kinship agency. While in the case of relatives in Vietnam the need for kinwork is concealed by the emphasis on the biogenetic, in the case of Czech grandmothers, kinwork is salient. In other words, the children explain their ties with Vietnamese grandmothers as done, permanent and based on common blood and genes. Contrary to this primordial definition, ties with Czech grandmothers tend to be described in terms of performativity—as negotiated, created and maintained in daily face-to-face contact. This strategy of relating themselves to a kinship network seems to be important for the children's sense of place in the world, which is marked by the duality and ambiguity between Czechness and Vietnameseness (see below). At the same time, this strategy provides children with a clue for understanding the delegated care-giving itself as well as its outcomes. It provides them with meaningful explanations of the differences in their ties with Czech grandmothers on the one side, and with parents and relatives in Vietnam on the other. The Czech grandma is an important reference point in the children's lives, connecting them to an older generation and to a new homeland. Intergenerational dependence often serves as grounds for socio-cultural dependency: the Czech grandma becomes the main anchor in the new society—a person who is trusted, and who spontaneously teaches the child "what life is like in the Czech Republic."

Socio-Cultural Dependency and Settlement through Nannies

All the mothers and nannies I interviewed understood child care—whether performed by mothers or nannies—as nurturance, and above all, as transmission of skills, and social and cultural capital (Macdonald, 2010; Bourdieu, 1986). The classic theory of social capital supposes that it is the "mother's task to transfer the abilities central to social capital to their children" (Kovalainen, 2004, p.167). Especially for migrant families, the role of parents and parental attitudes are likely to be important to their descendants' ethnic identity (Phinney *et al.*, 2001). In her study on Vietnamese immigrant families in the USA, Nazli Kibria (1993) shows how the postmigratory redefinition of family life goes hand in hand with the accentuation of Vietnamese cultural identity. "Vietnameseness"—maintained above all in the realm of family life—is the main point of reference helping immigrants to find a new place in the new country. For many mothers who delegate child care, the issue of how to transmit cultural and social capital as well as habitus through nannies "who may not naturally carry the same social and cultural assumptions" (Macdonald, 2010, p.26) becomes crucial. Motherhood is culturally and socially specific, and culture is actively transmitted through mothering. What if mothering is delegated from migrant mother to native nanny?

Ties based on sociocultural dependency are created during the coexistence of nannies and families from different socio-cultural backgrounds. Vietnamese children (and their parents) become the "windows to exotica" (Rollins, 1985) for the Czech nannies; and Czech nannies, analogically, are the "doors to majority" for Vietnamese children. In her book on domestic workers and their relationship with employers, Judith Rollins writes that in some cases employers use their domestic workers as so-called "windows to exotica" (Rollins, 1985, p.157 and p.166). The employee usually provides the employer with her only contact with a "third culture" (see also Anderson, 2000). This way the employee becomes a "window to exotica" for her employer when she mediates her the insight in her own—the third—culture. Rollins adds that in many cases the domestic worker provides confirmation of white middle-class women's stereotypes regarding "the Third World," and serves to justify a system which maintains certain types of persons in positions of disadvantage. The metaphor of "a window" is useful for portraying the experience of mutual socio-cultural dependency between nannies and families (especially children, but also to lesser extent parents). The "cultural exchange" between nannies and families is mutual, as each teaches something new about their culture. It is up to nannies, mothers, and children to decide which traits they will select and adopt into their lives and identities. This selection is more strictly done by nannies and mothers, as the children learn during their childhood how to strike a balance between Vietnameseness and Czechness.

The socio-cultural dependency of nannies on families can be described by the metaphor of the "window to exotica." Similarly to what Rollins describes, the Vietnamese child is usually the only (or at least the only very intensive) contact with "otherness" in the ethnically homogenous Czech society. As discussed in this book, the nannies react differently to children's physical otherness, which can be surmounted when the emotional ties develop between them and the child. The ethnic otherness of the mother, however—often articulated when reflecting on the mothers' mothering—is stable and unchangeable. When taking care of a Vietnamese child, the Czech nannies get in touch with a culture of "the other." This may include "ethnic food"—exotic fruits, or a Vietnamese spring roll—which is served to nannies, or particular pieces of Vietnamese culture which the nannies can observe in Vietnamese families' households—for example Vietnamese altars for ancestors.

To capture the dependency of children on nannies I use the metaphor of the "door to majority" (see also Souralová, 2014). While Vietnamese families provide their nannies a look at "exotic" Vietnamese culture (hence the "window"), Czech nannies offer Vietnamese children an entrance to the majority culture (hence "door"). Social dependency arises mainly when the nannies pass their own social capital on to the children, introducing them to their friends and relatives, and substituting the children for their own missing social network. Cultural dependency is most evident in the passing down of language skills and Czech traditions and customs. The children themselves say that thanks to their nanny, they are better integrated into Czech society. They recognize that even without their nannies they would of course have got to know about the Czech culture and habits by learning about it at school or observing it around them. However, thanks to their Czech nannies, these children could experience all of what they call "the Czech way of life"—including for example how to spend time at Christmas or Easter, how to go mushroom hunting, and what a pig-slaughtering is, etc. When nannies become grandmas that pass their social and cultural capital to their Vietnamese grandchildren, these nannies also transmit to the children a sense of belonging to a collective. As evident in Chapters 5 and 6, care-giving as the basis of kinship, and kinship as the basis of home-bonding, are essential parts of the imagination of homeland. Hence for many children, their Czech grandmothers become the main point of reference for children's feeling of belonging and understanding of their position in a country that is not their parents' country of origin.

The dependency between children and parents is much more complicated. On the one hand, the children are dependent on their parents when it comes to forming their own ethnic identity. Their parents are the most important "access points" to Vietnameseness. The parents do as much as possible to transmit Vietnamese ethnic identity to their children—pushing them to speak Vietnamese; talking about their childhood in Vietnam; planning visits to Vietnam; being in touch with relatives in Vietnam or having Vietnamese TV channels at home. Children find themselves under the ambivalent expectations of their parent, who want their children to integrate into Czech society while at the same time remaining (or more precisely becoming) Vietnamese. On the other hand, the parents are dependent on their children's Czech linguistic and cultural skills, learned from the nannies. As Chapter 4 showed, this parental dependency on the children often puts children in the role of adults in negotiating with offices and bureaucracies, and allows parents to invest less time and effort into their own societal integration.

* * *

In summary, and to answer the main question of *"What is the character of the relationships among mothers, nannies and children?,"* we must consider care-giving as a formative activity which establishes ties between mothers, nannies and children whose subjectivities are mutually shaped in the daily practice of care-giving. The ties between nannies and mothers are based on the logic of employment, and reflect the disagreements and tensions as to what constitutes good motherhood. The ties between children and mothers are created on the basis of biological relations, but must be performed and reaffirmed in the daily practice of caring. The mother becomes a mother when she mothers/cares for the child, while the child becomes the mother's child (meaning offspring) when he/she receives the mother's care. And finally, the ties between nannies and children are based on the mutual exchange of emotions and everyday care-giving, both of which lead to the establishment of kinship ties and the subjectivation of nannies to grandmothers and cared-for children to grandchildren.

* * *

In the interviews, I asked my child interviewees if they could imagine being parents and hiring a nanny for their children. This question was motivated by my awareness that children brought up by nannies may easily find themselves, as adults, in a similar situation to that of their parents. First, if they meet the high educational expectations of their parents, most of these children will become professionals, and probably live in dual-career households in the Czech Republic, where government support for child care facilities is quite poor. In other words, they will become the prototype of the private child care demanders, referred to in the mainstream scholarship. And second, if their parents really leave for Vietnam—as the children expect they will—these children, as adults, will not be able to rely on their parents to help with childrearing. (It is also questionable whether the children would want their parents to take care of their children, given their own parents do not speak Czech very well). Therefore, what were the children's responses to my question? Most of them replied that it would depend on their job, but that they definitely would not like to stay with children for the maximum, four-year family leave in the Czech Republic, which is also the age when it is possible to place a child in kindergarten; "I am not studying so hard now just to stay at home with kids later," was one of the most common answers. At the same time, they would not like to return to work before their child is at least two years old (so they would not like to follow the model of returning to work when the child is six months old, which many of their parents did). Hence in the coming years it will be interesting to observe the continuity in care-giving strategies, and look at how the future parents/former children brought up by Czech nannies make their care-giving decisions with reference to their own childhood experiences.

Appendices

A.1 Profiles of the study participants 1 (children)

child's pseudonym	gender	age[1]	place of birth/ age when coming to the CR
Minh	M	17	Czech Republic
Mia	F	16	Czech Republic
Anh	F	22	Vietnam, 5 years
Yen	F	19	Czech Republic
Hanh	F	18	Czech Republic
Danh	M	24	Vietnam
Lien	F	17	Czech Republic
Linh	F	19	Vietnam, 7 months
Thi	F	21	Vietnam, 5 years
Xuan	F	23	Vietnam, 7 years
Nguyet	F	21	Vietnam, 4 years
Tuyet	F	21	Vietnam, 3 years
Huynh	M	17	Czech Republic
Khanh	F	21	Vietnam, 4 years
Quyen	F	21	Vietnam, 6 years
Hue	F	20	Czech Republic
Han	F	17	Czech Republic
Kim	F	18	Vietnam, 5 years, previously living in Germany, now in CR
Bui	F	19	Czech Republic
Trai	M	25	Vietnam, 7 years

A.2 Profiles of the study participants 2 (mothers)

mother's pseudonym	number of children	year of arrival in the Czech Republic	caregiving/relationship at the time of being interviewed
Ms. Pham	1	2005	Caregiving
Ms. Truong	1	1991	Relationship
Ms. Tran	2	1993	Caregiving
Ms. Ngoc	2	1999	Caregiving
Ms. Ho	2	1996	Caregiving
Ms. Duong	2	1997	relationship
Ms. Ngo	3	1992	relationship
Ms. Ly	2	1998	Caregiving
Ms. Nguyen	2	1980	relationship
Ms. Do	2	2002	Caregiving
Ms. Ngo	1	1997	relationship
Ms. Phan	3	1993	relationship
Ms. Vu	2	1995	relationship
Ms. Dang	2	2000	Caregiving
Ms. Huynh	1	2002	Caregiving

A.3 Profiles of the study participants 3 (nannies)

nanny's pseudonym	position in welfare state	number of families	caregiving/relationship at the time of being interviewed
Ms. Špačková	parental leave	5	relationship
Ms. Brhlíková + her daughter Lenka Brhlíková	disability pensioner	1	caregiving
Ms. Křepelková	disability pensioner	5	caregiving
Ms. Kosová	pensioner	1	relationship
Ms. Zezulková	pensioner	1	caregiving
Ms. Orlová	pensioner	2	relationship
Ms. Dudková	pensioner	1	caregiving
Ms. Andulková	pensioner	1	relationship
Ms. Lelková	pensioner	1	relationship
Ms. Jestřábová	unemployed	2	caregiving
Ms. Zvonková	unemployed + care for husband	1	caregiving
Ms. Kolibříková	pensioner	1	caregiving
Ms. Havranová	pensioner	1	relationship
Ms. Rorýsová	employed	2	relationship
Ms. Čápová	unemployed	2	caregiving

Note: At the moment of conducting the interview.

Bibliography

Abel, E.K., Nelson, M.K., 1990. *Circles of Care.* Albany: State University of New York.

Akalin, A., 2007. Hired as a Caregiver, Demanded as a Housewife: Becoming a Migrant Domestic Worker in Turkey. *European Journal of Women's Studies*, 3(14), pp. 209–225.

Akalin, A., 2008. Turning Labour into Love: The Employment of Migrant Domestic Workers in Turkey. In: Sigrid Metz-Göckel, Mirjana Morokvašić-Müller, Agnes Senganata Münst (eds). *Migration and Mobility in an Enlarged Europe: A Gender Perspective*. Opladen: Barbara Budrich Publishers. pp. 103–120.

Andall, J., 2003. Hierarchies and Interdependence: The Emergence of a Service Caste in Europe. In: Jacqueline Andall (ed.). *Gender and Ethnicity in Contemporary Europe*. Oxford: Berg. pp. 39–60.

Anderson, B., 1983. *Imagined Communities: Reflections on the Origin and Spread of. Nationalism.* London: Verso.

Anderson, B., 2000. *Doing the Dirty Work? The Global Politics of Domestic Labour.* London and New York: Zed Books.

Anderson, B., 2003. Just Another Job? The Commodification of Domestic Labour. In: Barbara Ehrenreich, Arlie Russell Hochschild (eds). *Global Woman: Nannies, Maids, and Sex Workers in the New Economy*. New York: Metropolitan Books. pp. 104–114.

Apitzsch, U., 2007. Citizenship, New Migration and Gender Diversity in Europe. In: Erik Berggren, Branka Likic-Brboric, Gülay Toksöz, Nicos Trimikliniotis (eds). *International Migration, Informal Labour and Community: A Challenge for Europe*. Maastricht: Shaker Publishing. pp. 226–261.

Arendell, T., 2000. Conceiving and Investigating Motherhood: The Decade's Scholarship. *Journal of Marriage and Family*, 62, pp. 1190–1207.

Armenia, A.B., 2009. More than Motherhood: Reasons for Becoming a Family Day Care Worker. *Journal of Family Issues*, 30, pp. 554–574.

Bakan, A.B., Stasiulis, D., 1995. Making the Match: Domestic Placement Agencies and the Racialization of Women's Household Work. *Signs: Journal of Women in Culture and Society*, 20(2), pp. 303–335.

Baláž, V., Williams, A.M., 2007. Path-dependency and Path-creation Perspectives on Migration Trajectories: The Economic Experiences of Vietnamese Migrants in Slovakia. *International Migration*, 45(2), pp. 37–67.

Boehm, D.A., 2012. *Intimate Migrations. Gender, Family, and Illegality among Transnational Mexicans.* New York: New York University Press.

Bourdieu, P., 2001. The Forms of Capital. In: Mark Granovetter, Richard Swedberg, (eds). *The Sociology of Economic Life*. Boulder and Oxford: Westview Press. pp. 96–111.

Brouček, S. 2003. *Aktuální problémy adaptace vietnamského etnika v ČR*. Praha: Etnologický ústav AV ČR.

Búriková, Z., 2007. Motivácie au pair migrácie zo Slovenska. *Slovenský národopis*, 4, pp. 442–456.

Búriková, Z., Miller, D., 2010. *Au Pair.* Cambridge: Polity Press.

Carsten, J., 2004. *After Kinship.* Cambridge: Cambridge University Press.

Chamberlain, M., 1997. *Narratives of Exile and Return.* London: Macmillan.

Chamberlayne, P., King, A., 2000. *Cultures of Care: Biographies of Carers in Britain and the Two Germanies*. Bristol: The Policy Press.

Chang, G., 2000. *Disposable Domestics. Immigrant Women Workers in the Global Factory*. Cambridge: South End Press.

Colen, S., 1995. 'Like a Mother to Them': Stratified Reproduction and West Indian Childcare Workers and Employers in New York. In: Faye D. Ginsburg, Ryana Rapp (eds). *Conceiving the New World Order: The Global Politics of Reproduction.* Berkeley, CA: University of California Press. pp. 78–102.

Collins, P.H., 1993. The Meaning of Motherhood in Black Culture and Black Mother-Daughter Relationships. In: Patricia Bell-Scott (ed.). *Double Stitch: Black Women Write About Mothers and Daughters.* New York: HarperPerenial. pp. 42–60.

Collins, P.H., 1994. Shifting the Center: Race, Class, and Feminist Theorizing about Motherhood. In: Nakano Glenn, Evelyn, Grace Change, Linda Rennie Forcey (eds). *Mothering: Ideology, Experience and Agency.* New York: Routledge. pp. 45–65.

Collins, P.H., 2000. *Black Feminist Thought: Knowledge, Consciousness, and the Politics of Empowerment.* New York: Routledge.

Constable, N., 1997. Sexuality and Discipline among Filipina Domestic Workers in Hong Kong. *American Ethnologist*, 24, pp. 539–558.

Cox, R., 2006. *The Servant Problem: Paid Domestic Work in a Global Economy.* London: I.B. Tauris.

Cox, R., Watt, P., 2002. Globalization, Polarization and the Informal Sector; the Case of Paid Domestic Workers in London. *Area*, 34(1), pp. 39–47.

DeVault, M.L. 1991. *Feeding the Family: The Social Organization of Caring as Gendered Work.* Chicago: University of Chicago Press.

Di Leonardo, M. 1987. The Female World of Cards and Holidays: Women, Families, and the Work of Kinship. *Signs* 12(3): 440–53.

Dudová, R., Hašková, H., 2010. Diskurzy, instituce a praxe péče o děti do tří let ve francouzsko-české komparativní perspektivě. *Gender, rovné příležitosti, výzkum*, 12(2), pp. 36–47.

Ebaugh, H.R., Curry, M., 2000. Fictive Kin as Social Capital in New Immigrant Communities. *Sociological Perspectives*, 43(2), pp. 189–209.

Ehrenreich, B., Hochschild, A.R. 2003. Introduction. In: Barbara Ehrenreich, Arlie Russell Hochschild (eds). *Global Woman: Nannies, Maids, and Sex Workers in the New Economy*. New York: Metropolitan Books. pp. 1–13.

England, K., Stiell, B., 1997. 'They Think You're as Stupid as Your English Is': Constructing Foreign Domestic Workers in Toronto. *Environment and Planning*, 29(2), pp. 195–215.

England, P. 2005. Emerging Theories in Care Work. *Annual Review of Sociology*, 31(1), pp. 381–399.

Erel, U., 2009. *Migrant Women Transforming Citizenship.* London: Ashgate.

Espiritu, Y.L., 1994. The Intersection of Race, Ethnicity, and Class: The Multiple Identities of Second Generation Filipinos. *Identities*, 1(2–3), pp. 249–273.

Espiritu, Y.L., 2003. *Home Bound: Filipino American Lives Across Cultures, Communities and Countries*. Berkeley, CA: University of California Press.

Espiritu, Y.L., Tran, T., 2002. Viet Nam, Nu'óc Tôi (Vietnam, My Country): Vietnamese Americans and transnationalism. In: Peggy Levitt, Mary Waters (eds). *The Changing Face of Home.* New York: Russell Sage. pp. 367–398.

Ezzy, D., 2002. *Qualitative Analysis. Practice and Innovation.* London: Routledge.

Faubion, J.D. 2001. Introduction: Towards the Anthropology of the Ethnics of Kinship. In: James Faubion (ed.). *The Ethics of Kinship: Ethnographic Enquiries.* Lanham: Rowman & Littlefield. pp. 1–28.

Flick, U., 2009. *An Introduction to Qualitative Research.* London: Sage.

Foner, N., 1997. The Immigrant Family: Cultural Legacies and Cultural Changes. *International Migration Review*, 31(4), pp. 961–974.

Forsberg, L., 2009. *Involved Parenthood: Everyday Lives of Swedish Middle-Class Families.* Linköping: Tema barn, doktorsavhandling.

Freed, A.O., 1988. Interviewing through an Interpreter. *Social Work*, 33(4), pp. 315–319.

Gathorne-Hardy, J., 1972. *The Rise & Fall of the British Nanny.* London: Hodder & Stoughton.

Glenn, E.N., 1992. From Servitude to Service Work: Historical Continuities in the Racial Division of Paid Reproductive Labor. *Signs: Journal of Women in Culture and Society*, 18(1), pp. 1–43.

Glenn, E.N., 1994. Social Constructions of Mothering: A Thematic Overview. In: Evelyn Nakano Glenn, Grace Change, Linda Rennie Forcey (eds). *Mothering: Ideology, Experience, and Agency*. New York: Routledge. pp. 1–29.

Glenn, E.N., 2000. Creating a Caring Society. *Contemporary Sociology*, 1, pp. 84–94.

Guo, Z., 2014. *Young Children as Intercultural Mediators: Mandarin-speaking Chinese Families in Britain.* Bristol: Multilingual Matters.

Gregson, N., Lowe, M., 1994. *Servicing the Middle Classes: Class, Gender and Waged Domestic Labour in Contemporary Britain.* London and New York: Routledge.

Hammersley, M., Atkinson, P., 1995. *Ethnography. Principles in Practice.* London: Routledge.

Hardin, Carolyn. "My American Grandma": Theorizing Fictive Kinship and Affective Visibility in the Lives of Immigrant Elder Care Workers [online]. San Diego (CA): National Communication Association Annual Conference, 2008 [cit. 16.4.2014]. Dostupné z: http://citation.allacademic.com//meta/p_mla_apa_research_citation/2/5/6/7/0/pages256705/p256705-1.php.

Hašková, H., 2008. Kam směřuje česká společnost v oblasti denní péče o předškolní děti? In: Alena Křížková, Radka Dudová, Hana Hašková, Hana Maříková, Zuzana Uhde (eds). *Práce a péče: Proměny rodičovské v České republice a kontext rodinné politiky Evropské Unie.* Praha: SLON. pp. 51–70.

Hasmanová Marhánková, J., Štípková, M., 2014. Typologie prarodičovství v české společnosti – faktory ovlivňující zapojení prarodičů do péče o vnoučata. *Naše společnost* 12(1): 15–26.

Hays, S., 1996. *Cultural Contradictions of Motherhood.* New Haven: Yale University Press.

Hess, S. 2003. Transmigration of Eastern European Women as Transformation Strategy. Available at http://no-racism.net/article/144/. (last visited 10/03/2013).

Hess, S., Puckhaber, A., 2004. "Big Sisters" Are Better Servants?! Comments on the Booming Au Pair Business. *Feminist Review*, 77, pp. 65–78.

Hochschild, A.R., 1983. *The Managed Heart: Commercialization of Human Feeling.* Berkeley, CA: University of California Press.

Hochschild, A.R., 2000. Global Care Chains and Emotional Surplus Value. In: Will Hutton, Anthony Giddens (eds). *On the Edge: Living with Global Capitalism.* London: Jonathon Cape. pp 130–146

Hochschild, A.R., 2003. Love and Gold. In: Barbara Ehrenreich, Arlie Russell Hochschild (eds). *Global Woman: Nannies, Maids, and Sex Workers in the New Economy.* New York: Metropolitan Books. pp. 15–30.

Hofírek, O., Nekorjak, M., 2009. Vietnamští imigranti v českých velkoměstech – integrace přistěhovalců z Vietnamu (Vietnamese immigrants in Czech cities – integration of immigrants from Vietnam). In: Miroslava Rákoczyová, Robert Trbola (eds). *Sociální integrace přistěhovalců v České republice.* Praha: SLON. pp. 160–197.

Hollway, W., 2006. *The Capacity to Care: Gender and Ethical Subjectivity.* London: Routledge.

Hondagneu-Soleto, P. 1994. *Gendered Transition: Mexican Experiences of Immigration.* California: University of California Press.

Hondagneu-Sotelo, P., 2001. *Doméstica: Immigrant Workers Cleaning and Caring in the Shadows of Affluence.* California: University of California Press.

Hondagneu-Sotelo, P., Avila, E. 1997. "I'm here, but I'm there": The Meanings of Latina Transnational Motherhood. *Gender and Society*, 11(5), pp. 548–571.

Howell, S., 2003. Kinning: the Creation of Life Trajectories in Transnational Adoptive Families. *Journal of the Royal Anthropological Institute*, 9, pp. 465–484.

Isaksen, L.W. (ed.), 2010. *Global Care Work. Gender and Migration in Nordic Societies.* Lund: Nordic Academic Press.

Isaksen, L.W., Devi, U., Hochschild, A.R., 2008. Global Care Crisis. Mother and Child's Eye View. *Sociologia, Problemas e Práticas*, 56, pp. 61–83.

Jenks, C., 2004. Constructing Childhood Sociologically. In: Kehily, M.J. (ed.) An Introduction to Childhood Studies. Open University Press. pp. 77–95.

Kao, Grace. 1995. Asian Americans as Model Minorities? A Look at their Academic Performance. *American Journal of Education*, 103(2), 121–59.

Karner, Tracy X. 1998. Professional caring: Homecare workers as fictive kin. *Journal of Aging Studies*, 12(1), 69–82.

Kibria, N., 1993. *Family Tightrope: The Changing Lives of Vietnamese Americans*. Princeton: Princeton University Press.

Kibria, N., 2005. Of Blood, Belonging, and Homeland Trips: Transnationalism and Identity among Second Generation Chinese and Korean Americans. In: Peggy Levitt, Mary Waters (eds). *The Changing Face of Home.* New York: Russell Sage. pp. 295–311.

King, R., Christou, A., Teerling, J. 2011. 'We Took a Bath with the Chickens': Memories of Childhood Visits to the Homeland by Second-Generation Greek and Greek Cypriot Returnee. *Global Networks*, 11(1), pp. 1–23.

Kovalainen, A., 2004. Rethinking the Revival of Social Capital and Trust in Social Theory: Possibilities for Feminist Analysis. In: Barbara Marshall, Anne Witz (eds). *Engendering the Social: Feminist Encounters with Sociological Theory*. Maidenhead: Open University Press. pp. 155–170.

Lan, P.C., 2002. Among Women: Filipina Domestics and their Taiwanese Employers across Generations. In: Barbara Ehrenreich, Arlie Russell Hochschild (eds). *Global Woman: Nannies, Maids, and Sex Workers in the New Economy.* New York: Metropolitan. pp. 169–189.

Lan, P.C., 2003. Negotiating Social Boundaries and Private Zones: the Micropolitics of Employing Migrant Domestic Workers. *Social Problems*, 50, pp. 525–549.

Lan, P.C., 2006. *Global Cinderellas: Migrant Domestics and Newly Rich Employers in Taiwan.* Duke: Duke University Press.

Lee, H., 2011. Rethinking Transnationalism through the Second Generation. *The Australian Journal of Anthropology*, 22(3), pp. 295–313.

Levitt, P., 2002. The Ties That Change: Relations to the Ancestral Home over the Life Cycle. In: Peggy Levitt, Mary Waters (eds). *The Changing Face of Home: The Transnational Lives of the Second Generation:* New York: Russell Sage Foundation. pp. 123–144.

Levitt, P., Waters, M.P., 2002. *The Changing Face of Home: The Transnational Lives of the Second Generation.* New York: Russell Sage Foundation.

Liamputtong, P. 2006. Motherhood and "Moral Career": Discourses of Good Motherhood Among Southeast Asian Immigrant Women in Australia. *Quantitative Sociology*, 29(1), pp. 25–53.

Lister, R. et al., 2007. *Gendering Citizenship in Western Europe: New Challenges for Citizenship Research in a Cross-National Context*. Bristol: Policy Press.

Lutz, H., 2008a. (ed.), *Migration and Domestic Work; A European Perspective on a Global Theme*. Aldershot: Ashgate.

Lutz, H., 2008b. Introduction: Migrant Domestic Work in Europe. In: Helma Lutz (ed.). *Migration and Domestic Work: A European Perspective on a Global Theme*. Aldershot: Ashgate. pp. 1–10.

Lutz, H., 2008c. When Home Becomes a Workplace: Domestic Work as an Ordinary Job in Germany? In: Helma Lutz (ed.). *Migration and Domestic Work; A European Perspective on a Global Theme*. Aldershot: Ashgate. pp. 43–60.

Lutz, H., 2011. *The New Maids. Transnational Women and the Care Economy*. London, New York: Zed Books.

Macdonald, C.L., 1998. Manufacturing Motherhood: The Shadow Work of Nannies and Au Pairs. *Qualitative Sociology*, 21(1), pp. 25–53.

Macdonald, C.L., 2010. *Shadow Mothers. Nannies, Au Pairs, and the Micropolitics of Mothering*. Berkeley, Los Angeles, London: University of California Press.

Madianou, M., Miller, D., 2011. *Migration and New Media: Transnational Families and Polymedia*. New York: Routledge.

Marjorie Faulstich Orellana, Lisa Dorner and Lucila Pulido. 2003. Accessing assets: Immigrant youth's work as family translators or "para-phrasers." *Social Problems*, 50(4), pp. 505–24.

Maroufof, Michaela. 2013. With All the Cares in the World: Irregular Migrant Domestic Workers in Greece. In: Triandafyllidou, Anna (ed.). *Irregular Migrant Domestic Workers in Europe: Who Cares?* Aldershot: Ashgate. p. 95–115.

Martínková, Š., 2006. Česko-vietnamské vztahy. In: Jiří Kocourek, Eva Pechová (eds). *S vietnamskými dětmi na českých školách*. Praha: H & H. pp. 84–93.

Matthews, H., Ewen, D. 2006. *Reaching All Children? Understanding Early Care and Education Participation Among Immigrant Families*. Center for Law and Social Policy. Available at: http://www.clasp.org/resources-and-publications/files/0267.pdf.

Mauss, M. 1990 (1922). *The Gift: Forms and Functions of Exchange in Archaic Societies*. London: Routledge.

McMahon, M., 1995. *Engendering Motherhood: Identity and Self-Transformation in Women's Lives*. New York: Guilford Press.

Momsen, J.H., 1999. *Gender, Migration and Domestic Service*. London: Routledge.

Moon, S., 2003. Immigration and Mothering: Two Generations of Middle-Class Korean Immigrant Women. *Gender & Society*, 17(6), pp. 840–860.

Morokvasic, M. 2004. 'Settled in Mobility': Engendering Post-Wall Migration in Europe. *Feminist Review*, 77, 7–25

Murray, S.B., 1998. Child Care Work: Intimacy in the Shadows of Family-Life. *Qualitative Sociology*, 2, pp. 149–168.

Nelson, M.K., 1989. Negotiated Care: Relationships between Family Daycare Providers and Mothers. *Feminist Studies*, 15(1), pp. 7–33.

Nelson, M.K., 1990. *Negotiated Care: The Experience of Family Day Care Providers*. Philadelphia: Temple University Press.

Nelson, M.K., 1994. Family Day Care Providers: Dilemmas of Daily Practice. In: Evelyn Nakano Glenn, et al. (eds). *Mothering: Ideology, Experience, and Agency*. New York: Routledge. pp. 181–209.

Nguyen, Huong, 2012. Child Care/Family Leave Policies in Vietnam. Available at: http://www.sjsu.edu/people/amy.d'andrade/courses/scwk202/s6/PPT%20Family%20Leave%20and%20Child%20Care%20FULL.pdf. (last visited 10/12/2012).

Oakley, A., 1974. *Woman's Work: The Housewife, Past and Present.* New York: Random House.

Oropesa, R.S., Landale, N.S., 1997. In: Search of the New Second Generation: Alternative Strategies for Identifying Second-Generation Children and Understanding Their Acquisition of English. *Sociological Perspectives*, 40(3), pp. 427–455.

Palmer, P.M., 1990. *Domesticity and Dirt. Housewives and Domestic Servants in the United States, 1920-1945.* Philadelphia: Temple University Press.

Parreñas, R.S., 2000. Migrant Filipina Domestic Workers and the International Division of Reproductive Labor. *Gender and Society*, 14(4), pp. 560–580.

Parreñas, R.S., 2001. *Servants of Globalization: Women, Migration, and Domestic Work.* Stanford, CA: Stanford University Press.

Parreñas, R.S., 2005. *Children of Global Migration: Transnational Families and Gendered Woes*. Stanford, CA: Stanford University Press.

Patton, M.Q., 1990. *Qualitative Evaluation and Research Methods*. Newbury Park, California: Sage.

Phinney, Jean S. et al. 2001. The role of language, parents, and peers in ethnic identity among adolescents in immigrant families, *Journal of Youth and Adolescence*, 30(2), p. 135–53.

Prout, A., James, A., 1997. A New Paradigm for the Sociology of Childhood. In: Alan Prout, Alison James (eds), *Constructing and Reconstructing Childhood.* London: Routledge/ Falmer. pp. 7–33.

Qvortrup, J., 1993. Nine Theses about "Childhood as a Social Phenomenon. In: *Childhood as a Social Phenomenon: Lessons from an International Project, Eurosocial Report 47/1993.* Vienna: European Center for Social Welfare Training and Research.

Rollins, J., 1985. *Between Women: Domestics and Their Employers.* Philadelphia: Temple University Press.

Romero, M., 1992. *Maid in the USA.* London and New York: Routledge.

Romero, M., 1997. Who Takes Care of the Maid's Children? Exploring the Costs of Domestic Service. In: Hilde Lindeman Nelson (ed.). *Feminism and Families.* New York, NY: Routledge. pp. 151–169.

Rumbaut, R.G., 2002. Severed or Sustained Attachments? Language, Identity, and Imagined Communities in the Post-Immigrant Generation." In: Peggy Levitt, Mary Waters (eds). *The Changing Face of Home: The Transnational Lives of the Second Generation.* New York: Russell Sage Foundation. pp. 43–95.

Rushdie, S., 1992. *Imaginary Homelands*. London: Penguin.

Ryan, L., 2007. Migrant Women, Social Networks and Motherhood: The Experiences of Irish Nurses in Britain. *Sociology*, 41(2), pp. 295–312.

Sahlins, M., 1985. *Islands of History*. Chicago: University of Chicago Press.

Sahlins, M., 2011. What Kinship Is (Part One). *Journal of the Royal Anthropological Institute*, 17(1), pp. 2–19.

Said, E. 1984. Reflections on Exile. *Granta*, 13, pp. 158–172.

Sarti, R. 2014. Historians, Social Scientists, Servants, and Domestic Workers: Fifty Years of Research on Domestic and Care Work. *International Review of Social History* 59(2), 279–314.

Schneider, D.M., 1984. *A Critique of the Study of Kinship*. University of Michigan Press: Ann Arbor.

Segura, D.A., 1994. Working at Motherhood: Chicana and Mexican Immigrant Mothers and Employment. In: Evelyn Nakano Glenn, Grace Change, Linda Rennie Forcey (eds). *Mothering: Ideology, Experience, and Agency*. New York: Routledge. pp. 211–233.

Simon, S., 1996. *Gender in Translation: Cultural Identity and the Politics of Transmission*. London: Routledge.

Sirovátka, T., Saxonberg, S., 2006. Failing Family Policy in Post-Communist Central Europe. *Journal of Comparative Policy Analysis*, 8(2), pp. 189–206.

Šlesingerová, E., 2014. *Imaginace genů. Sociologická perspektiva*. Praha: SLON.

Šlesingerová, E., 2005. Imaginace genů a hranice etnických identifikací. *Sociální studia*, 2, pp. 35–55.

Šmausová, G., 2002. Proti tvrdošíjné představě o ontické povaze genderu a pohlaví. *Sociální studia*, 7, pp. 15–27.

Song, M., 1999. *Helping Out. Children's Labor in Ethnic Businesses*. Philadelphia: Temple University Press.

Souralová, A. 2015. Mutual Emotional Relations in Caregiving Work at the Turn to the Twenty-First Century: Vietnamese Families and Czech Nannies-Grandmothers. In: Dirk Hoerder, Elise van Nederveen Meerkerk, Silke Neunsinger. *Towards a Global History of Domestic and Caregiving Workers*. Leiden: Brill. pp. 182–201.

Souralová, A., 2014a. Vietnamese Immigrants in the Czech Republic: Hiring a Czech Nanny as a Post-Migratory Family Settlement Strategy. In: Sylvia Hahn, Stan Nadel. *Asian Migrants in Europe. Transcultural Connections*. Göttingen: Vandenhoeck & Ruprecht V&R unipress. pp. 95–112.

Souralová, A., 2014b. The Czech Nanny as a 'Door to the Majority' for Children of Vietnamese Immigrants in the Czech Republic. *Studia Migracyjne – Przegląd Polonijny*, 40(3), pp. 171–186.

Temple, B., Edwards, R., 2002. Interpreters/Translators and Cross Language Research: Reflexivity and Border Crossings. *International Journal of Qualitative Methods*, 1(2), pp. 1–11.

Tilly, C., Brown, H.C., 1967. On Uprooting, Kinship, and the Auspices of Migration. *International Journal of Comparative Sociology*, 8, pp. 139–164.

Tronto, J.C., 2002. The 'Nanny' Question in Feminism. *Hypatia*, 1(2), pp. 31–51.

Uttal, L., 1996. Custodial Care, Surrogate Care, Coordinated Care: The Meaning of Child Care to Employed Mothers. *Gender & Society*, 10(3), pp. 291–311.

Uttal, L., 1999. Using Kin for Child Care: Embedment in Family Socioeconomic Webs. *Journal of Marriage and the Family*, 61(4), pp. 845–857.

Uttal, L., Tuominen, M., 1999. Tenuous Relationships. Exploitation, Emotion, and Racial Ethnic Significance in Paid Child Care Work. *Gender and Society*, 13(6), pp. 758–780.

Wall, K., José, J.S., 2004. Managing Work and Care: A Difficult Challenge for Immigrant Families. *Social Policy & Administration*, 38(6), pp. 591–621.

Walzer, S., 1997. Contextualizing the Employment Decisions of New Mothers. *Qualitative Sociology*, 20(2), pp. 211–227.

Wessendorf, S., 2007. Roots-Migrants: Transnationalism and "Return" among Second-Generation Italians in Switzerland. *Journal of Ethnic and Migration Studies*, 33(7), pp. 1083–1102.

Williams, A.M., Baláž, V., 2004. From Private to Public Sphere, the Commodification of the Au Pair Experience? Returned Migrants from Slovakia to the UK. *Environment and Planning*, 36, pp. 1813–1833.

Williams, A.M., Baláž. V., 2005. Winning, then Losing, the Battle with Globalisation: Vietnamese Petty Traders in Slovakia. *International Journal of Urban and Regional Research*, 29(3), pp. 533–549.

Wolf, D.L., 2002. There's no Place Like "Home": Emotional Transnationalism and the Struggles of Second-Generation Filipinos. In: Peggy Levitt, Mary C. Waters (eds). *The Changing Face of Home: The Transnational Lives of the Second Generation.* New York: Russell Sage Foundation. pp. 255–294.

Wrigley, J., 1995. *Other People's Children. An Intimate Account of the Dilemmas Facing Middle-Class Parents and the Women they Hire to Raise their Children.* New York: Basic Books.

Wrigley, J., 1999. Hiring a Nanny: The Limits of Private Solutions to Public Problems. *Annals of the American Academy of Political and Social Science*, 563(1), pp. 162–174.

Wu, F., 2002. *Yellow: Race in America beyond Black and White.* New York: Basic Books.

Yuval-Davis, N., 2011. *The Politics of Belonging. Intersectional Contestations.* London: Sage.

Resources

www.czso.cz (Czech Statistical Office)
www.cssz.cz (Czech Social Security Administration)
www.mpsv.cz (Ministry of Labour and Social Affairs)
www.szu.cz (Institute of Health Information and Statistics of the Czech Republic)

Index

For Product Safety Concerns and Information please contact our EU representative GPSR@taylorandfrancis.com
Taylor & Francis Verlag GmbH, Kaufingerstraße 24, 80331 München, Germany

www.ingramcontent.com/pod-product-compliance
Lightning Source LLC
Chambersburg PA
CBHW060744150926
51501CB00003B/90
9781472456663